PRESCRIBING IN PREGNANCY

Third edition

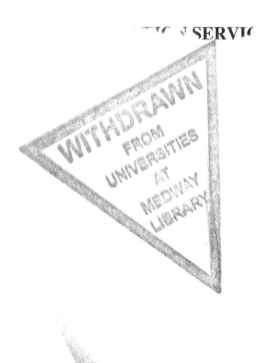

PRESCRIBING IN PREGNANCY

Third edition

Edited by

PETER RUBIN

Professor, Department of Medicine,
Queen's Medical Centre, Nottingham, UK

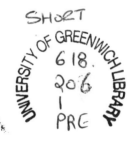
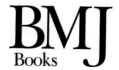

BMJ
Books

© BMJ Books 2000
BMJ Books is an imprint of the BMJ Publishing Group

First published in 1987
by the BMJ Publishing Group, BMA House, Tavistock Square,
London WC1H 9JR

www.bmjbooks.com

First edition 1987
Second edition 1995
Third edition 2000
Second impression 2002

British Library Cataloguing in Publication Data
A catalogue record for this book is available from the British Library

ISBN 0-7279-1449-9 $\mathcal{SRB}$

Typeset by J&L Composition Ltd, Filey, North Yorkshire
Printed and bound by Selwood Printing Ltd. West Sussex

Contents

CONTENTS

Contributors

Anthony J Avery
Senior Lecturer, Division of General Practice, The Medical School, Queen's Medical Centre, Nottingham, UK

Margaret A Byron
Consultant and Honorary Senior Lecturer in Rheumatology, University of Bristol Division of Medicine, Rheumatology Unit, Bristol Royal Infirmary, Bristol, UK

Kate Campbell
Diabetes Nurse Specialist, Diabetes Centre, Royal Sussex County Hospital, Brighton, East Sussex, UK

Susan Carr
Senior Pharmacist, Leicestershire Drug Information Service, Leicester Royal Infirmary, Leicester, UK

Michael de Swiet
Consultant Physician, Institute of Obstetrics and Gynaecology, Imperial College School of Medicine, Queen Charlotte's and Chelsea Hospital, London, UK

Bill Hague
Consultant Physician in Obstetric Medicine, Women's and Children's Hospital, Clinical Senior Lecturer in Obstetrics, Department of Obstetrics, University of Adelaide, South Australia

Mary Hepburn
Senior Lecturer in Women's Reproductive Health, Department of Obstetrics and Gynaecology and of Social Policy and Social Work, Glasgow Royal Maternity Hospital, Glasgow, UK

Helen E Hopkinson
Lecturer, Division of Therapeutics, Department of Medicine, Queen's Medical Centre, Nottingham, UK

CONTRIBUTORS

Pauline A Hurley
Consultant Obstetrics/Fetal Medicine, The Women's Centre,
John Radcliffe Hospital, Oxford, UK

Lena M Macara
Consultant Obstetrician & Gynaecologist, The Queen Mother's
Hospital, Glasgow, UK

Catherine Nelson-Piercy
Consultant Obstetric Physician, Guys and St. Thomas' Hospitals Trust,
Department of Obstetrics, St. Thomas' Hospital, 7th Floor, North Wing,
London, UK

Kevin Nicholls
Consultant Psychiatrist, Shelton Hospital, Bicton Heath, Shrewsbury,
UK

Peter Rubin
Professor, Department of Medicine, Queen's Medical Centre,
Nottingham, UK

Jane M Rutherford
Specialist Registrar, Division of Feto-maternal Medicine, Queen's
Medical Centre, Nottingham, UK

Guy Sawle
Reader in Clinical Neurology, Queen's Medical Centre, Nottingham,
UK

Nick Vaughan
Consultant Diabetologist, Diabetes Centre, Royal Sussex County
Hospital, Brighton, East Sussex, UK

Timothy MA Weller
Consultant Microbiologist, Department of Microbiology, City Hospital,
Birmingham, UK

Richard Wise
Professor, Department of Medical Microbiology, City Hospital,
Birmingham, UK

Catherine Williamson
Honorary Senior Registrar in Obstetric Medicine, Maternal and Fetal
Disease Group, Clinical Research Building, Hammersmith Hospital,
London, UK

Preface

The use of drugs in women who are pregnant or breast feeding is a question of fine balance. Harm may befall a baby because a drug has been used, but mother and baby could suffer if a disease goes untreated. Information about the safe and effective use of drugs in pregnancy has not kept pace with the advances in other areas of therapeutics. Systematic research involving drugs in pregnancy is fraught with ethical, legal, emotional and practical difficulties and in many cases our knowledge is based on anecdote or small studies.

The purpose of this book is to bring together what is known about prescribing in pregnancy and to put that information in a clinical context. The first two editions were well received and this has encouraged us to produce a third edition. All chapters have been extensively revised or rewritten, with several new authors bringing their clinical experience of this challenging subject.

I am particularly grateful to my personal assistant, Louise Sabir, for her considerable help in the preparation of this book and to Mary Banks and her colleagues at the BMJ for their continued encouragement.

Peter Rubin
Nottingham

1 Identifying fetal abnormalities

LENA M MACARA

Key points

- Day 18–55 post conception is the time of maximal teratogenic potential while tissues/organs are differentiating.

- Teratogenic effects may affect organ development and/or organ function.

- Detailed ultrasound scanning will detect major structural abnormalities, but many "minor" defects may not be seen with current machinery.

- Patients at risk of neural tube defects have 5 mg folic acid for at least 6 weeks prior to conception.

Introduction

Over the last few decades, the range of medicinal products available on a prescribed basis and for sale, both illicitly and as "over the counter preparations", has expanded enormously. When drugs are taken during pregnancy, there are always majors concerns that the baby will be permanently damaged. Whilst over 2% of all pregnancies in the United Kingdom are affected by congenital abnormalities, over 50% of these are of unknown aetiology. A further 25% may be linked to a variety of genetic problems, and only 2% are likely to be associated with drugs. However, the problem of drug use in pregnancy is not small. One prospective Finnish study demonstrated that 12% of women use analgesics during pregnancy, and up to 9% were on regular prescribed medication,

1

usually for chronic disease such as asthma, hypertension, and thyroid disease.[1] The National Institute on Drug Abuse (NIDA) National Health and Pregnancy survey in 1992 also confirmed extensive use of medication during pregnancy, with almost 6% of pregnant women in the United States using illicit drugs, 20% using alcohol and/or nicotine, and over 10% on psychotherapeutic drugs such as sedatives, tranquillizers, or analgesics during pregnancy.[2]

The vast majority of patients who take medicinal preparations during pregnancy do not have an increased risk of fetal abnormalities, and reassurance is all that is required. Sometimes, however, teratogenicity is a real possibility and identifying this group is difficult. This chapter aims to guide clinicians faced with women who have conceived while on treatment, in order to identify those who would benefit from additional obstetric and/or paediatric input.

Embryonic and fetal development

It is clear from practice that not all drugs affect a pregnancy in an identical manner or to the same degree of severity. This is due to the rapid but staggered sequence of events which occurs as two cells multiply to form the embryo and fetus that we recognize. Understanding the order and timing of this process may help us both to understand which organ systems are likely to be affected at each stage of pregnancy and anticipate the possible long-term effects which may ensue.

Fetal development can be divided into three main stages:

- the *predifferentiation or pre-embryonic phase*, from conception until 17 days post conception
- the *embryonic stage* from 3 to 8 weeks post conception; and
- the *fetal phase* from week 8 until term.

During the predifferentiation stage, the cells of the conceptus divide rapidly and remain totipotent. Any insult to the pregnancy during this phase seems to have an "all or nothing" effect. If most of the cells are affected, the pregnancy is spontaneously miscarried but when only some cells are affected, the remaining totipotent cells appear to replace the damaged cells without any long-term deleterious effect. Most women will not yet have missed their first period and therefore may not realize they are pregnant.

During the embryonic period, these cells differentiate and form definitive organ systems (Figure 1.1) Since the cells have differen-

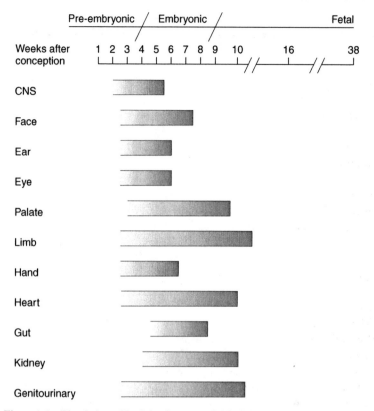

Figure 1.1 The timing of fetal development. Critical time periods of development for each organ system.

tiated, once damaged they are unlikely to be replaced and permanent effects are likely to ensue. Although the embryonic period is short, each end organ has a window of maximal susceptibility, when the organ is forming and teratogenic insults are likely to be most severe. In some circumstances, the effects seen are dosage dependent.

The fetal period is primarily a time of growth and maturation, and most drugs are therefore unlikely to cause structural defects. However, organs such as the cerebral cortex and renal glomeruli continue to differentiate and remain vulnerable to growth or functional damage.

The type and degree of teratogenic effects seen in pregnancy is determined by the stage of development when exposure occurs. Establishing the gestational age of the pregnant woman at presentation and the stage at which the medication was taken will confirm if there is any potential risk to the pregnancy. The clinician must then confirm if the medication taken has any known teratogenic risks.

Potential teratogenic compounds

The United States Food and Drug Administration (FDA) categorized all drugs into five main groups from A (safe to use in pregnancy) through to D (contraindicated in pregnancy) and X for extremely toxic drugs, which should never be used in pregnancy.[3] However, these are only guidelines and should not form the basis on which risks of teratogenesis are assessed and termination of pregnancy is offered. Some drugs are commonly used, often of necessity, during pregnancy and are summarized below. Later chapters give a more detailed description of these drugs and their place in pregnancy therapy.

Antibiotics

Penicillins and cephalosporins do not seem to be teratogenic.[4] In the case of antituberculous drugs, ethambutol, and isoniazid have a good safety record but streptomycin causes deafness. Rifampicin, which causes neural tube defects (NTD) and facial clefting in mice,[5] is associated with a human fetal abnormality rate two or three times higher than ethambutol or isoniazid but is still within the expected range. Ethionamide has been associated with exomphalos and exencephaly, and should be avoided.

Table 1.1 Drugs commonly used in pregnancy with known teratogenic profiles

Drug group	Teratogenic profile	Risks of teratogenesis
Hydantoins	craniofacial abnormalities, mental retardation, NTD	~6%
Valproate	NTD, microcephaly	~2% risk of NTD
Carbamazepine	NTD, craniofacial	~6%
Warfarin	CNS problems, bone stippling, craniofacial abnormalities	Up to 25% risk of abnormality if exposure in first 6 weeks (but disputed – see Chapter 4)
Lithium	cardiac defects	2%
Retinoids	CNS, CVS, craniofacial	High

Anticonvulsants

All the long-established anticonvulsant therapies are associated with teratogenic effects. Overall there is a two- to four-fold increase in the incidence of malformations in babies of epileptic mothers.[6] These fall into three main groups: namely central nervous system (CNS), cardiovascular (CVS), and craniofacial abnormalities. Hydantoins are associated with a variety of craniofacial (cleft lip, flat nose, hypterelorism) and limb defects (hypoplasia of distal phalanges) in particular, which together are known as the hydantoin syndrome. Up to 10% of fetuses exposed to hydantoins will be affected by the syndrome which unfortunately is neither dose- nor duration of use-related. In addition, one-third of these neonates will have more severe defects such as microcephaly. Whilst craniofacial defects are also seen with sodium valproate and carbamazepine, there are additional risks of neural tube defects (NTD) with valproate that in part appear to be dose-related. The defects seen are usually of the spina bifida variety rather than the lethal, anencephaly end of the spectrum.[7] Little is known about newer anticonvulsants.

Anticonvulsants may affect vitamin K-dependent clotting factors. Oral vitamin K supplements should be given to mothers for at least 1 week prior to delivery to reduce the risks of neonatal bleeding.[8]

Anticoagulants

Both heparins and warfarin are used during pregnancy. To date there have been no adverse fetal effects documented with heparin as neither unfractionated nor low molecular heparins cross the placenta. Since 1975, a number of recognized abnormalities have been associated with warfarin use.[9] Facial defects, such as nasal hypoplasia and stippling of the long bones, are common. In addition, complex anomalies of the central nervous system such as microcephaly and Dandy–Walker malformations may be seen. Even in the absence of these abnormalities, significant mental retardation may occur. It is estimated that 25–30% of babies exposed to warfarin in the first trimester, particularly during weeks 6–12, can be affected.[10]

Antihypertensives

There are no reported fetal abnormalities with most of the drugs used in cardiovascular disease therapy. Angiotensin-converting enzyme inhibitors (ACEI) cross the placenta and can cause fetal anuria and hypotension.[11] Although there are reported cases successfully managed with ACEI,[12] the effects may not be reversible at delivery or following cessation of treatment, and these drugs should not be used during the 2nd and 3rd trimesters.

Psychotropic drugs

Tricyclic antidepressants are not associated with fetal abnormalities and although fluoxetine has been linked with perinatal complications by some,[13] specific fetal abnormalities have not been identified. Fluoxetine has been widely used by others with no adverse outcomes reported.[14] Benzodiazepines have been linked with craniofacial abnormalities, particularly cleft palate, but this is still disputed. Lithium is associated with specific fetal abnormalities, mainly cardiac defects. Ebstein's anomaly, in which the tricuspid valve is distorted and displaced, has been reported in about one-third of affected babies, although coarctation of the aorta and valve atresias can also be seen.[15] A detailed fetal cardiac scan at 20 weeks' gestation should be offered to all women on lithium treatment.

Dermatological preparations

Retinoic acid is contraindicated in pregnancy because 25% of babies will be affected by congenital abnormalities. Craniofacial defects, CNS, and CVS defects have all been reported. While CNS defects predominate, up to one-third will have cardiovascular problems.[16] After long-term treatment, clearance of the drug is reduced. Teratogenic effects may still be seen for some time after stopping treatment, and patients should therefore avoid pregnancy for at least 1 year.[17]

Analgesics

Non-steroidal anti-inflammatory (NSAI) drugs should be avoided in pregnancy, although they are sometimes used, of necessity, to suppress preterm labour. When they are used for prolonged periods of time or in a high dosage, fetal urine production is impaired and may not recover following delivery. As most of these effects are mediated through the cyclo-oxygenase 1 (cox-1) pathways, new selective cox-2 NSAI drugs may not have the same risk profile.

Pregnancy management

Ideally pregnancy management should commence in the pre-conception period and all drug therapy carefully evaluated. Where possible, polypharmacy should be reduced to a minimum and drugs with the least teratogenic profile used. Those using medication associated with risks of NTD, such as anticonvulsants, should be commenced on 5 mg folic acid for at least 6 weeks prior to conception to minimize the risks of NTD developing.[18,19] Folic acid may also reduce the risks of facial clefting in patients on anticonvulsant therapy.[20]

From these discussions it is clear that some teratogenic effects are structural and some functional. High resolution detailed ultrasound scanning by experienced personnel is recommended to detect structural problems, but functional defects cannot be detected antenatally unless they cause other problems which may be noted on scan. It is important to recognize that, whilst major abnormalities should always be identified, many more minor defects, such as cleft lip and palate, may not be noted, even in referral centres. Moreover, dysmorphic features or flatting of facial bones will not be seen on most standard ultrasound scans. The main anomalies likely to be detected antenatally are outlined below

Central nervous system

Anencephaly should be detected by 12 weeks' gestation, when a biparietal diameter is not clearly visualized. Spina bifida is more subtle and is often not detected on ultrasound until 16–18 weeks gestation. Maternal serum screening with alpha-fetoprotein is routinely offered in most units between 15 and 21 weeks' gestation, and patients are recalled for a detailed scan if the level is elevated above two multiples of the median. With this regimen, only 85% of NTD will be identified and, for patients at increased risk of NTD, this is not sufficient. Patients in this category, for example those on anticonvulsant therapy, should routinely be offered a detailed scan, irrespective of the alpha-fetoprotein. Where normal views of the fetal spine and intracranial anatomy are seen (Figures 1.2, 1.3), the patient should be reassured. Up to 80% of babies with an NTD will have intracranial signs due to an Arnold–Chiari type malformation, namely an abnormal cerebellum and hydrocephalus (Figures 1.4, 1.5). Amniocentesis, to detect the acetylcholinesterase band specific for NTD, should only be required when there is difficulty in obtaining satisfactory views of the spine, as there is a 1% risk of miscarriage with the procedure. Where an NTD is identified, the parents should be counselled, and offered the option of talking to a paediatric surgeon. Women who choose to continue with the pregnancy should be delivered in a tertiary unit to ensure

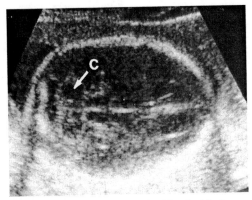

Figure 1.2   Ultrasound image of a normal fetal head with the cerebellum clearly seen.

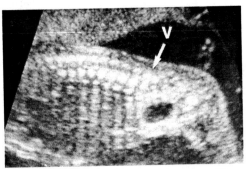

Figure 1.3   A normal fetal spine with the lower sacral vertebrae (V) merging in a point.

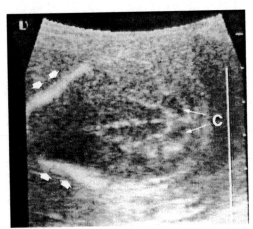

Figure 1.4   Arnold–Chiari type malformation in a baby with spina bifida, showing the abnormal cerebellum (C) and indrawing of the frontal bones (arrow heads).

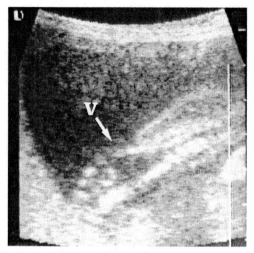

Figure 1.5   Fetal spina bifida on ultrasound with splaying of the fetal vertebrae (V).

minimal damage to any exposed neural tissue at the time of delivery and early paediatric intervention.

Other abnormalities, such as Dandy–Walker type malformations (Figure 1.6) and cerebral cysts, may be detected antenatally. As the outlook for these babies is very variable and depends on the presence or absence of other abnormalities, referral to a specialist unit is recommended.

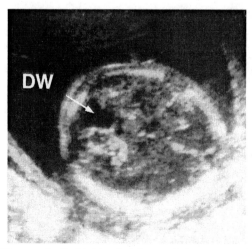

Figure 1.6   Ultrasound of a fetal head. A large echolucent area (Dandy–Walker [DW] type malformation) is present in the posterior fossa.

Cardiovascular system (CVS)

Fetal cardiology is a relatively recent development reflecting the recent improvements in imaging. While it was initially hoped that nearly all abnormalities could be detected, experience has taught that even in specialist units only 70–80% are likely to be identified antenatally, and detection rates as low as 20% have been reported.[21,22] When a normal four-chamber view of the heart is seen (Figure 1.7), up to 40% of anomalies are excluded. In women at risk of CVS anomalies, the outflow tracts should also be identified, to eliminate defects such as Fallot's tetralogy. Many cardiac defects are seen in association with chromosome abnormalities and fetal karyotyping may therefore be advisable before allowing the pregnancy to continue. Since the management and prognosis for cardiac defects are constantly changing, referral to a unit with paediatric cardiology on site is advised. Many babies with cardiac defects also benefit from delivery in a specialist unit and early intervention.

Facial clefting

This is one of the commonest abnormalities associated with teratogenesis. Although large complete mid-line defects are readily recognized (Figure 1.8), isolated cleft palate and small unilateral cleft lips can easily be missed. A "normal" facial profile will exclude major defects. Since this problem can be very distressing for

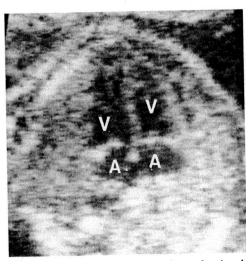

Figure 1.7. A normal four-chamber view of the heart showing the ventricles (V) and atria (A).

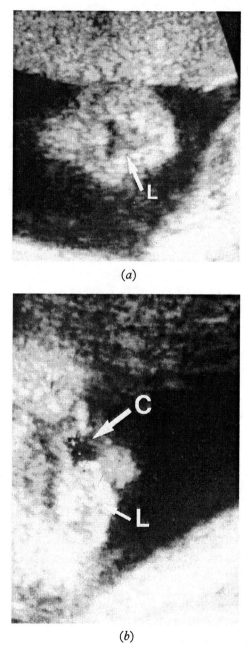

(a)

(b)

Figure 1.8   (a) Normal profile of fetal lips (L) in the second trimester. (b) Profile of fetal lips showing the upper lips (L) with a large cleft (C) present.

parents, antenatal referral to a local cleft palate team can help parents to prepare prior to delivery. Staged corrective surgery with excellent long-term results are possible in affected children. Other craniofacial abnormalities, such as hypertelorism or a thin upper lip, cannot be identified with current scan imaging. The new three-dimensional scan systems being introduced to clinical practice may well prove useful in the future for detecting these "minor" soft markers, since the actual facial profile can be clearly visualized.

Skeletal problems

It is relatively easy to measure fetal limbs during pregnancy, but many subtle deviations in growth do not present until the third trimester, well beyond the time of detailed anomaly scanning. Gross defects of the type associated with thalidomide should easily be detected by 18 weeks. Where teratogenesis is suspected, careful inspection of the hands, feet, and digits should be made. Other aetiologies for skeletal problems are common and should be excluded before any defects are attributed to drug ingestion. Reconstructive surgery and limb replacement is often possible in childhood.

Functional defects which may be detected antenatally

During the second half of pregnancy amniotic fluid is derived almost exclusively from fetal urine. The effects of drugs on the kidney may therefore be detected antenatally. There are many other causes for reduced liquor, such as poor placental function, obstruction in the renal tract, and spontaneous rupture of the membranes, so a drug effect is often a diagnosis of exclusion and may not be confirmed until after delivery. The main drugs known to have this effect are ACE inhibitors and prostaglandin synthase inhibitors.

Fetal behavioural patterns have been noted to be altered in sheep with cocaine use, but these are currently research tools rather than diagnostic criteria to predict fetal and neonatal outcome. Cocaine use is also strongly associated with poor placental function.[23] This cannot be tested antenatally, although poor placental function usually results in poor fetal growth, and this can be evaluated by ultrasound.

Summary

Most congenital abnormalities are not related to drug use in pregnancy. Where drugs are known to cause structural abnormalities, detailed ultrasound scans in the second trimester can be used to confirm or exclude a problem. When an abnormality is detected, the parents have the option of termination of the pregnancy where the problem is substantial, or planned delivery when early paediatric input is beneficial. Detailed ultrasound scans cannot detect functional abnormalities, such as mental retardation, or minor problems, such as dysmorphic features. In the event of this being detected at birth, other common causes of mental retardation must be excluded before a specific drug is blamed. It is prudent for all clinicians presented with a woman, who has used medication during pregnancy, to ensure careful documentation at the time of presentation, as many functional problems are often not identified until the child is several months old, and recollecting the timing of drug exposure and the investigations performed can be difficult at a later date.

References

1 Heillila AM, Erkkola RU, Nummi SE. Use of medication during pregnancy – a cohort study on use and policy of prescribing. *Annls Chirurg Gynaecolog* 1994; **83** (Suppl. 208): 80–3.

2 Mathias R. NIDA Survey provides first national data on drug use during pregnancy. *Nat Ins Drug Abuse Notes* 1995; **10**: http://www.nida.nih.gov

3 United States Food and Drug Administration. Labelling and prescription drug advertising. Content and format for labelling for human prescription drugs. *Fed Reg* 1979; **44**: 434–67.

4 Greenberg G, Inman WHW, Weatherall JAC, Adelstein AN, Haskey JC. Maternal drug histories and congenital abnormalities. *BMJ* 1977; **ii**: 853–6.

5 Steen JSM, Stainton-Ellis DM. Rifampicin in pregnancy. *Lancet* 1977; **2**: 604–5.

6 Lindhout D, Omtzigt JGC. Teratogenic effects of antiepileptic drugs: implications for the management of epilepsy in women of childbearing age. *Epilepsia* 1994; **35** (Suppl. 4): S19–28.

7 Samren EB, van Duijn CM, Koch S *et al.* Maternal use of anti-epileptic drugs and the risks of major congenital malformations. A joint European prospective study of human teratogenesis associated with maternal epilepsy. *Epilepsia* 1997; **38**: 981–90.

8 Thorp JA, Gaston L, Caspers DR, Pal MA. Current concepts and controversies in the use of vitamin K. *Drugs* 1995; **49**: 376–7.

9 Pettifor JM, Benson R. Congenital malformations associated with the administration of oral anti-coagulants during pregnancy. *J Paediat* 1975; **86**: 459–62.

10 Iturbe-Alessio I, del Carmen Fonseca M, Mutchinik O, Santos MA, Zajanas A, Salazar E. Risks of anticoagulant therapy in pregnant women with artificial heart valves. *New Engl J Med* 1986; **315**: 1390–3.

11 Rosa FW, Bosco LA, Fossum-Graham C, Milstein JB, Dreis M, Creamer J. Neonatal anuria with maternal angiotesin converting enzyme inhibitor. *Obstet Gynecol* 1989; **74**: 371–4.

12 Kreft-Jais C, Plouin C, Tchobroutsky C, Boutroy MJ. Angiotensin converting enzyme inhibitors during pregnancy: A survey of 22 patients given captopril and 9 given enalapril. *Br J Obstet Gynaecol* 1988; **95**: 420–2.

13 Chambers CD, Johnson KA, Dick LM, Felix RJ, Jones KL. Birth outcomes in pregnant women taking Fluoxetine. *New Engl J Med* 1996; **335**: 1010–15.

14 Pastuszak A, Schick-Boschetto B, Zuber C *et al.* Pregnancy outcome following first trimester exposure to fluoxetine (prozac). *JAMA* 1993; **269**: 2246–8.

15 Cohen LS, Freidman JM, Jefferson JW, Johnson EM, Weiner ML. A re-evaluation of of risk of in-utero exposure to lithium. *JAMA* 1994; **271**: 146–50.

16 Lammer EJ, Chen DT, Hoar RM. Retinoic acid embryopathy. *New Engl J Med* 1985; **313**: 837–41.

17 Cordero AA, Allerato MA, Donatti L. Ro-10-9359 and pregnancy. In: *Retinoids: advances in basic research and therapy*. Berlin: Springer, 1981, p. 501.

18 Reynolds EH. Anti-convulsants, folic acid and epilepsy. *Lancet* 1973; **1**: 1376–88.

19 MRC Vitamin Research Study Group. Prevention of neural tube defects: results of the MRC vitamin study. *Lancet* 1991; **338**: 131–9.

20 Shaw GM, Lammer EJ, Wasserman CR, O'Malley CD, Tolarova MM. Risks of oro-facial clefts in children born to women using multivitamins containing folic acid periconceprtionally. *Lancet* 1995; **346**: 399.

21 Allan LD. Echocardiographic detection of congenital heart disease in the fetus: present and future. *Br Heart J* 1995; **74**: 103–6.

22 Eik-Nes SH, Tegnander E. Fetal heart screening: a diagnostic challange. In: *The fetus as a patient* (Eds. Chervenak FA, Kurjak A). New York: Parthenon Publishing 1996, pp. 147–58.

23 Woods JR(Jr), Plessinger MA, Clark KE. Effect of cocaine upon uterine artery blood flow and fetal oxygen. *JAMA* 1987; **257**: 957–61.

2 Treatment of common minor and self-limiting conditions

ANTHONY J AVERY, SUSAN CARR

Key points

- Where possible, try non-drug treatments first.
- In selecting drugs:
  - choose the one that has the best safety record over time;
  - avoid newer drugs, unless safety has been clearly established;
  - don't assume that over-the-counter drugs and herbal medicines are safe.
- In deciding on doses and treatment courses:
  - avoid the first 10 weeks of gestation if possible;
  - use the lowest effective dose;
  - use the drug for the shortest period of time necessary;
  - where possible, use drugs intermittently rather than continuously.

Introduction

This chapter deals with the management of some common and self-limiting conditions that may occur during pregnancy. Since most of these are minor, non-drug treatments should be used whenever possible.

In this chapter we discuss drugs in pregnancy for the following:

- symptoms affecting the gastrointestinal tract;
- minor ailments involving the respiratory tract;

15

- short-term painful conditions;
- common fungal infections;
- common infestations.

A summary of the drugs discussed under each of these headings is given in Table 2.1.

Table 2.1 Drugs used for common minor and self-limiting conditions, and their safety in pregnancy

Refer to text before using this table. Use any drug in lowest possible dose for shortest time.

Condition and drug	Manufacturers advice	Trimester 1	Trimester 2	Trimester 3	Comment
Nausea & Vomiting					
cyclizine		1	1	1	
promethazine		1	1	1	
metoclopramide		1	1	1	
domperidone	A	1	1	1	
prochlorperazine		1	1	1	
Gastrointestinal					
antacids		1	1	1	
alginate-antacids, e.g. Gaviscon, Algicon		1	1	1	
cimetidine	A	1	1	1	
ranitidine		1	1	1	
omeprazole		2	2	2	
lactulose		1	1	1	
senna		2	2	2	
bisacodyl		2	2	2	
docusate		2	2	2	
glycerin suppositories		1	1	1	
loperamide	A	2	2	2	
co-phenotrope		2	2	2	
Respiratory					
topical sympathomimetics e.g. xylometazoline		1	1	1	
intranasal corticosteroids		1	1	1	
antitussives, e.g. codeine		2	1	2	
dextromethorphan		2	2	2	
pholcodine		2	2	2	
sodium cromoglycate drops		1	1	1	
beclomethasone nasal spray		1	1	1	
chlorpheniramine		1	1	1	
promethazine		1	1	1	
terfenadine		2	2	2	
cetirizine	A	2	2	2	
loratadine	A	2	2	2	
Pain					
paracetamol		1	1	1	
aspirin		2	2	2	
NSAIDs		2	1	3	Ibuprofen preferred
opioids including morphine, pethidine, fentanyl, hydromorphone, oxycodone		1	1	2	Newborn may be opioid dependent
co-proxamol		3	2	2	
sumatriptan		3	3	3	
ergotamine		3	3	3	
Common fungal infections					
clotrimazole (topical)		1	1	1	Nystatin less effective than clotrimazole
nystatin (topical)		1	1	1	
fluconazole	A	2	2	2	
ketoconazole	A	3	3	3	Avoid high dose/regular use
itraconazole	A	3	3	3	
griseofulvin	A	3	3	3	
terbinafine		3	3	3	

Table 2.1 *continued*

Common infestations					
malathion		1	1	1	Aqueous
permethrin		1	1	1	preparation
phenothrin		1	1	1	preferable
carbaryl		2	2	2	
piperazine	A	2	1	1	
mebendazole	A	2	1	1	

Key: 1 = drug probably safe during pregnancy; 2 = safety uncertain, or insufficient data; 3 = unsafe, or very limited experience; A = manufacturer advises avoid during pregnancy.

The gastrointestinal tract

Nausea and vomiting

A substantial proportion of women suffer from nausea, vomiting, or both during the early stages of pregnancy, typically between 6 and 12 weeks' gestation. Although known colloquially as "morning sickness" the symptoms can occur at any time of the day. The cause is poorly understood, although thought to be related to raised levels of human chorionic gonadotrophin (HCG). Most women who suffer symptoms of nausea and vomiting manage to limit these by avoiding foods likely to exacerbate symptoms, and eating at times of the day when symptoms are less severe. Simple advice such as eating smaller meals which are high in carbohydrate and low in fat, and avoidance of large volumes of fluid (substituting smaller volumes more frequently) may be helpful.

More severe vomiting may occur in a minority of women and can lead to dehydration, ketosis, and weight loss, requiring admission to hospital. If nausea and vomiting are severe, drug treatment may be justified. Controlled trials have not been done, and there is little evidence of comparative efficacy of drugs in relieving symptoms. However, there are data available for outcome following use of some antiemetic drugs. One meta-analysis of 24 studies involving over 200 000 women exposed mainly to antihistamines concluded that there was no increased risk of teratogenicity associated with use of such drugs.[1] A number of other drugs including the dopamine antagonists metoclopramide and domperidone have been used, as has the phenothiazine, prochlorperazine. These have not been associated with a teratogenic effect, although the studies have involved smaller numbers of women than with the antihistamines.[2] In selecting a drug for treating nausea and vomiting in pregnancy, it is reasonable to try one of the older sedative antihistamines first, as these have probably had the widest use.

17

Alternative therapies, including powdered root of ginger, have been shown to be effective in hyperemesis[3], and acupressure was effective in relieving nausea but not vomiting.[4] We are not aware of any controlled studies of morning sickness using homeopathic remedies.

Gastro-oesophageal reflux and heartburn

Gastro-oesophageal reflux and heartburn are reported by a substantial proportion of women throughout pregnancy and are caused by a fall in lower oesophageal sphincter pressure, which is probably related to rising levels of progesterone.[5,6] Symptoms are similar to those that occur in the non-pregnant state. Conservative measures such as avoiding late meals in the evening or before retiring, raising the head of the bed by 10–15 cm, and avoiding fatty or strongly spiced foods may be helpful.

Antacids containing calcium, magnesium, or aluminium may be useful and are generally considered safe.[7] Similarly, preparations containing alginates (Gaviscon®, Algicon®) are largely not absorbed and considered safe to use. Sucralfate is a mucosal protective agent which is not absorbed in significant amounts. It is based on aluminium hydroxide and has been shown to be effective in relieving heartburn and regurgitation during pregnancy.[8]

Histamine H2–blocking drugs are frequently used to treat gastro-oesophageal reflux in non-pregnant patients. Data from animal studies and anecdotal reports in humans are reassuring about the use of these drugs in pregnancy, although a possible anti-androgen effect has been identified in rats given cimetidine.[9] However, there are no large prospective studies and it is probably appropriate to use these agents only in patients with severe and persistent symptoms which do not respond to the lifestyle changes or treatments outlined above. Experience with cimetidine and ranitidine has been more extensive than with famotidine or nizatidine, and for this reason the former two drugs are probably preferable.[10]

Proton pump inhibitors have become widely used in the treatment of gastro-oesophageal reflux in recent years. Animal toxicity studies have shown increased embryo and fetal mortality in rats and rabbits given doses of omeprazole far in excess of those administered to humans.[10] A recent prospective study of 113 women who took omeprazole during the period of organogenesis found no increased incidence of major malformations over a control group.[11] However, there have been several reports of anencephaly.[12] Less information is available for lansoprazole. Although it has not been shown to have teratogenic effects in animal reproductive studies,[13] we are not aware of any published reports on outcomes in human pregnancies.

Constipation

Constipation in pregnancy is common. Rising levels of progesterone affect gut motility, and this may be exacerbated by dietary changes, particularly during the early stages when nausea and/or vomiting is prominent. Consumption of iron preparations and aluminium-containing antacids may also contribute to symptoms. Principles of treatment of constipation are similar to those in the non-pregnant state. First-line treatment should involve increasing the intake of fruit (dried as well as fresh) and vegetables. Fluid intake should also be increased. Bulking agents such as ispaghula (e.g. Fybogel®, Regulan®) taken with plenty of fluid may be helpful. Lactulose is not appreciably absorbed and may also be helpful, although there is no extensive literature to support its use. Stimulant drugs including senna and bisacodyl are probably best avoided. Although senna is not thought to be teratogenic,[12] and we are not aware of any such published data for bisacodyl, these drugs may stimulate uterine contractions in the third trimester,[14] and are best avoided. Docusate sodium has not been linked to specific congenital defects although there are insufficient data to be able to recommend its use in pregnancy. Purgatives containing magnesium or sodium salts as the principal ingredient may cause electrolyte disturbances and are best avoided. Glycerol (glycerin) suppositories are unlikely to have adverse affects on the fetus.

Diarrhoea

Diarrhoea during pregnancy has similar causes to that in the non-pregnant patient, and should be investigated according to the presenting symptoms and signs. Gastroenteritis is the most common cause of diarrhoea in the child-bearing years and is usually self-limiting. Treatment should be aimed at maintaining hydration, using rehydration solution if necessary. Use of antidiarrhoeal drugs is best avoided as experience is limited. Diphenoxylate with atropine (co-phenotrope; Lomotil®) has not been found to be teratogenic in animals; one study reported no malformations in seven infants exposed during the first trimester.[15] Although there is a report suggesting problems with this combination in humans,[16] the timing of administration was not consistent with defects found.

19

Although loperamide is not thought to be teratogenic in animals,[17] we have seen no published studies and experience is limited.[12]

Haemorrhoids

Although many adults suffer with haemorrhoids, they are particularly common in pregnancy. Treatment is similar to that in the non-pregnant individual: avoidance of constipation, and use of a bland astringent cream if necessary.

Upper respiratory tract

Upper respiratory tract infections (URTIs) and hayfever are common problems for women of child-bearing age. Below we discuss the appropriateness of using antimicrobial agents in URTI. We then comment on the safety of drugs used for symptomatic treatment of upper respiratory problems.

In patients with symptoms of the "common cold", research suggests that there is no indication for using antibiotics.[18] However, that group of patients who have pathogenic bacteria in their nasopharyngeal secretions may benefit from treatment.[19] If sinusitis develops, most studies suggest that antibiotics reduce the duration of symptoms, and therefore their use may be justified.[20,21] Nevertheless, one well-conducted study showed no benefit from antibiotics,[22] and one should remember that most patients will make a full recovery from sinusitis whether they receive antibiotics or not. This may influence treatment choices in pregnancy.

A meta-analysis of studies involving the treatment of sore throat with antimicrobial agents suggests that treatment confers only modest benefits.[23] For example, the duration of symptoms is shortened by a mean of half a day at the time of maximal effect, and by approximately eight hours overall. There is probably a decreased risk of glomerulonephritis with antibiotic treatment.[23] However, the incidence of this complication is so low in Western societies that it is difficult to justify the use of antibiotics for this reason alone.

Overall, we would suggest not prescribing antibiotics for pregnant women with upper respiratory tract infections, unless symptoms are particularly distressing. For patients with tonsillitis it may be worth getting a throat swab before deciding whether to treat.

Symptomatic treatments for common upper respiratory problems

Given that the treatment of upper respiratory tract infections is essentially symptomatic, it is important to focus on the safety of preparations available. Over-the-counter preparations for colds contain a diversity of ingredients. Frequently the principal ingredient is paracetamol or aspirin. (See section below on Analgesics for more details of these drugs.) Other ingredients may include sympathomimetics, antihistamines, non-steroidal anti-inflammatory agents, and/or stimulants such as caffeine. Preparations with a multiplicity of ingredients are best avoided, and it is probably safest to give paracetamol alone if a drug is needed for pyrexia or malaise. Sympathomimetics may help with early symptoms of nasal congestion, but they have diminished effect over time and may cause rebound congestion. Nose drops (e.g. xylometazoline) are preferable to systemic preparations if treatment is seen to be necessary. If a woman wishes to use a particular favourite cold remedy, its safety should be checked with the manufacturer: ingredients in such preparations may change from time to time without notice.

Cough suppressants

Weak opioids such as codeine, pholcodine or dextromethorphan are often used as cough suppressants. Although they can partially suppress the cough reflex, they are not particularly effective and they are rarely essential for the treatment of URTIs. Surveillance studies on the use of codeine in pregnancy have not differentiated between the low doses used in cough suppressants and higher analgesic doses. Several published studies have identified a possible increase in malformations associated with the use of codeine,[15,24,25] and in one of these studies there was a statistically significant increase in respiratory malformations associated with the use of the drug.[15] In the other studies, there was an increased number of malformations, although this was not attributable to one particular defect.[24,25]

Another report identified symptoms of opioid withdrawal in two infants whose mothers had regularly taken codeine-containing cough mixtures late in pregnancy, although the mothers did not experience symptoms.[26] There are fewer published data for pholcodine and dextromethorphan. We suggest that opioid cough suppressants should be avoided during pregnancy, particularly during the first and third trimesters. If used, they should be taken intermittently rather than continuously and only if symptoms are severe – for example, if a cough is seriously interfering with sleep.

Expectorants are generally considered ineffective and therefore there is little point in using them. Similarly, preparations such as simple linctus have no influence on the cough mechanism. Nevertheless, simple linctus may be soothing, and it might be worth trying before giving pharmacological treatment.

Hayfever

Hayfever may be problematic for some women during pregnancy. Avoidance of the precipitating allergen, if known, can reduce the need for medication. Topical treatments should generally be tried before systemic therapy in order to reduce exposure of the fetus to drugs. Sodium cromoglycate eye drops are considered to be safe as the systemic dose is very small.[27]

Topical corticosteroid preparations in nasal sprays may be used for rhinitis, but systemic steroids should not be necessary, and there is no indication for depot injections.[28]

Topical sympathomimetics have been discussed above. The problem with using these in hayfever is that prolonged use may cause rebound nasal congestion.

If a systemic antihistamine is considered essential, older sedating agents such as chlorpheniramine or promethazine are preferable to the newer non-sedating agents on the grounds of more extensive safety data.[29] Terfenadine has been used during pregnancy, although the Michigan Medicaid project identified an excess of children with polydactyly where the mother had been exposed to this drug during the first trimester.[12] Insufficient data are currently available to assess the safety of cetirizine and loratadine in pregnancy, although they have not been identified as teratogens in animals.[29]

Pain and the use of analgesics in pregnancy

Paracetamol

Paracetamol has been used widely at all stages in pregnancy for relief of pain and as an antipyretic. Its short-term use during pregnancy has not been associated with congenital defects when taken in normal therapeutic doses. One study of women in the 1970s found that 41% had used paracetamol during the first half of their pregnancy.[30]

Aspirin

Aspirin is also taken widely in pregnancy, with one estimate suggesting that about 60% of pregnant women take the drug at some point.[31] In high doses, aspirin has been shown to be teratogenic in animal studies, while there is controversy about the risk in human pregnancy.[32] However, aspirin certainly does have a number of undesirable actions in the pregnant woman, principally in late pregnancy. In analgesic doses, it increases the risk of maternal or neonatal bleeding by virtue of its antiplatelet effect.[33] Also, it may delay the onset of labour and increase its duration.[34] For these reasons, analgesic doses of aspirin are best avoided in pregnancy, particularly in the third trimester.

Non-steroidal anti-inflammatory drugs (NSAIDs)

NSAIDs inhibit prostaglandin synthesis in a wide range of tissues, including the gut, the kidneys, platelets, and sites of inflammation. Their ability to cause premature closure of the ductus arteriosus at term has been recognized for many years, but they can also lead to renal dysfunction, intracerebral haemorrhage, and necrotizing enterocolitis in the newborn if given from around 24 weeks' gestation.[35]

NSAIDs are best avoided in pregnancy if at all possible.

Opioid analgesics

Much of the data relating to the safety of opioid analgesics in pregnancy has been gathered from studies of women misusing opioids. Such substances are often adulterated and opiate misusers may inadvertently use mixtures with other drugs. Two American surveillance projects (Michigan Medicaid and Collaborative Perinatal Project) have not recorded an excess rate of congenital defects associated with the use of morphine, pethidine, fentanyl, hydromorphone, oxycodone, or methadone.[12] Codeine use has been associated with an excess of respiratory malformations (see discussion of "Cough suppressants" above). Also, a possible association of congenital abnormalities with propoxyphene (an ingredient of co-proxamol in the UK) has been identified.[12]

Common fungal infections

Candida

Vaginal infections with *Candida* spp. are a common cause of discomfort during pregnancy. Topical agents such as clotrimazole, that have low systemic absorption, are considered to be without significant risk. A recent systematic review of treatment of vaginal candidiasis in pregnancy concluded that imidazoles such as clotri-mazole and econazole were more effective than nystatin and that the optimum duration of therapy was one week.[36] Systemic treatment is probably less desirable. There have been reports of congenital malformations in women who took regular doses of oral fluconazole in the first trimester of pregnancy for ongoing fungal infections such as coccoidomycosis.[37] There are fewer data available on exposure to intermittent or single dose use of the drug, as is likely for vaginal candidiasis. One prescription event monitoring study recorded the outcome of pregnancy in women who had taken either a single 150 mg dose of fluconazole (275 women), several 50 mg doses (three women) or multiple 150 mg doses (11 women) either during or shortly before becoming pregnant.[38] No abnormalities were identified in those who had taken fluconazole in early pregnancy. Another prospective study concluded that exposure to single doses or short courses of fluconazole during the first trimester did not appear to increase the incidence of congenital defect.[39] Although these data are reassuring, fluconazole is clearly best avoided during pregnancy. Itraconazole and ketoconazole are chemically related to fluconazole and also taken by mouth. Several reports have linked these drugs to congenital malformations,[12] and they should also be avoided.

Fungal skin infections

Topical imidazoles, such as clotrimazole, can be used to treat most ringworm infections including tinea pedis. For nail and scalp infections, systemic treatment with drugs such as griseofulvin and terbinafine may be required. However, on current evidence, these drugs should be avoided in pregnancy. Griseofulvin has been found to be both embryotoxic and teratogenic in some animal species,[12] and the manufacturer notes that it has been associated with some abnormalities in humans.[40] As damage to germ cells has been noted, there is an additional recommendation that men should not father children within six months of treatment with this drug.[40] Terbinafine is a more recently introduced antifungal agent. Animal studies have not found adverse effects on the fetus.[41] The manufacturer (Novartis, personal communication) has information on the outcomes of 44 pregnancies in women who had taken terbinafine during pregnancy. Excluding miscarriages (eight) and terminations of pregnancy (six), there were 30 live births. Of these, there were two deaths: one in a premature baby; a child with Patau syndrome/trisomy 13, and one in a child with a minor degree of hypospadias. While these events appeared not to have been related to terbinafine, we would suggest avoiding the drug in pregnancy unless absolutely necessary.

Common infestations

Headlice and threadworms are two infestations which women with school age children may find difficult to control. Also, scabies is not uncommon in young adults. These conditions are discussed below.

Head lice

Head lice (*Pediculus capitis*) have a life cycle of some 40 days, although the infestation has often been established for several months before being detected. The usual treatment involves topical application of one of four insecticides: phenothrin, permethrin, malathion, or carbaryl. However, combing with a fine-toothed comb has also been found to be effective (for details see Livingstone[42]).

Some health authorities in the UK have a rotational policy for head lice treatments in order to try to minimize the development of resistance. While this may influence drug choice in some locations, it is important to consider the most appropriate choices in pregnancy:

- Aqueous topical preparations are preferable to alcoholic formulations because systemic absorption may be lower, although this may reduce ovicidal activity.
- While it may be tempting to use insecticide shampoos to reduce the risks of systemic absorption, the short contact time means that they are relatively ineffective.[43]
- There are specific concerns about some of the drugs used for treating head lice. For example, in 1995 the use of carbaryl was restricted to prescription-only use in the UK because of worries about carcinogenicity from studies where rats were exposed to large doses over their lifespan. Lindane (no longer available in the UK) is unsuitable for use during pregnancy due to systemic absorption, followed by storage in body fat, and subsequent transfer to the infant during breastfeeding.[43]

The drug of choice in treating head lice in pregnancy is malathion, because there has been more experience with this drug than with newer preparations. If an insecticide is used in a pregnant woman, intensive combing with a detection comb for 1–2 weeks after treatment may help avoid re-infestation from lice which hatch from eggs unaffected by treatment. This may help avoid a subsequent course of treatment.

Scabies

Scabies (*Sarcoptes scabiei*) are parasites that burrow under the skin and cause intense pruritis, which is often worse at night. They are spread by close personal contact. Many of the drugs used for head lice are effective against scabies. However, given the considerations outlined above, the treatment of choice in pregnancy is an aqueous preparation of malathion. This should be applied topically to the whole body, excluding the head and neck. Pruritis takes some time to resolve after treatment, and therefore a sedative antihistamine, such as chlorpheniramine, may be helpful at night.

Threadworms

Threadworms (*Enterobius vermicularis*) develop in the gastrointestinal tract from ingested eggs. Female worms may then emerge onto the perianal skin to lay eggs, often at night. Pruritis occurs and scratching of the area allows eggs to be transferred to the fingernails. Re-infestation, or spread to other people, may then occur. Non-pharmacological treatment involves hygiene measures aimed to break the cycle of re-infestation. These include a bath or shower in the morning to remove eggs, scrubbing nails, strict handwashing before handling food, frequent changing of bed linen and wearing of close fitting pants at night. This is the most desirable method of controlling the problem in pregnant women, particularly in the first trimester of pregnancy. Other members of the household can be treated at the same time with anthelmintics.

Simple hygiene measures sometimes prove ineffective, and medication may be necessary if the worms are causing significant problems with pruritis. Unfortunately, data relating to safety of the two commonly used agents, mebendazole and piperazine, are relatively sparse. Mebendazole is known to be teratogenic in rats, but not in a number of other species.[44] However, it is only poorly absorbed from the gastrointestinal tract. Piperazine has not been reported to be teratogenic in animals, but it is systemically absorbed to a greater extent than mebendazole. Two anecdotal reports have sought to associate use of piperazine with congenital abnormalities.[45] Although the use of either mebendazole or piperazine is best

26

avoided in the first trimester, women who have taken these drugs inadvertently may be reassured that the risks to the fetus are low.[45]

References

1 Seto A, Einarson T, Koren G. Pregnancy outcome following first trimester exposure to antihistamines – metaanalysis. *Am J Perinatol* 1997; **14**: 119–24.

2 Nelson-Piercy C Treatment of nausea and vomiting. *Drug Safety* 1998; **19**: 155–64.

3 Fischer-Rasmussen W, Kjaer S K, Dahl C *et al.* Ginger treatment of hyperemesis gravidarum. *Am J Obstet Gynecol Repro Biol* 1991; **38**: 19–24.

4 Belluomini J, Litt R C, Lee KA *et al.* Acupressure for nausea and vomiting of pregnancy: a randomized, blinded study. *Obstet Gynecol* 1994; **84**: 245–8.

5 Baron TH, Ramirez B, Richter JE. Gastrointestinal motility disorders during pregnancy. *Ann Intern Med* 1993; **118**: 366–75.

6 Van Thiel D H, Gavaler J S, Stremple J. Heartburn of pregnancy. *Gastroenterology* 1977; **72**: 666–8.

7 Lewis JH, Weingold AB. The committee on FDA related matters, American College of Gastroenterology. *Am J Gastroenterol* 1985; **80**: 912–23.

8 Ranchet G, Gangemi O, Petrone M. Sucralfate in the treatment of gravidic pyrosis. *G Ital Osterica Ginecol* 1990; **12**: 1–16.

9 Parker S Schade RR, Pohl CR *et al.* Prenatal and neonatal exposure of male rat pups to cimetidine but not ranitidine adversely affects subsequent adult sexual functioning. *Gastroenterology* 1984; **86**: 675–80.

10 Broussard CN, Richter JE. Treating gastro-oesophageal reflux disease during pregnancy and lactation: What are the safest therapy options? *Drug Safety* 1998; **19**: 325–37.

11 Lalkin A, Loebstein R Addis R, Ramezani-Namin F *et al.* The safety of omeprazole during pregnancy: A multicenter prospective controlled study. *Am J Obstet Gynecol* 1998; b: 727–30.

12 Briggs GG, Freeman RK, Yaffe SJ. *Drugs in pregnancy and lactation.* Baltimore/London: Williams & Wilkins, 5th edn, 1998.

13 Wyeth pharmaceuticals. Data sheet for Zoton® (lansoprazole). In: *ABPI Compendium of data sheets and summaries of product characteristics 1998–9.* London: Datapharm Publications, 1998.

14 Lee A, Schofield S. Drug use in pregnancy: (2) Common medical problems. *Pharm J* 1994; **252**: 57–60.

15 Heinonen OP, Slone D, Shapiro S. *Birth defects and drugs in pregnancy.* Littleton MA: Publishing Sciences Group, 1977.

16 Siebert JR Barr M Jr Jackson JC Benjamin DR. Ebsteins anomaly and extracardiac effects. *Am J Dis Child* 1989; **143**: 570–2.

17 Janssen-Cilag. Data sheet for Imodium® (loperamide). In: *ABPI Compendium of data sheets and summaries of product characteristics 1998–9.* London: Datapharm Publications, 1998.

18 Arroll B, Kenealy T. Antibiotics versus placebo in the common cold (Cochrane Review). In: *The Cochrane Library,* Issue 1 1999. Oxford: Update Software, 1999.

19 Kaiser L, Lew D, Hirschel B *et al.* Effects of antibiotic prescribing in the subset of common-cold patients who have bacteria in their nasopharyngeal secretions. *Lancet* 1996; **347**: 1507–10.

20 Lindbaek M, Hjortdahl P, Johnsen UL. Randomised, double blind, placebo controlled trial of penicillin V and amoxycillin in treatment of acute sinus infections in adults. *BMJ* 1996; **313**: 325–9.

21 Low DE, Desrosiers M, McSherry J *et al.* A practical guide for the diagnosis and treatment of acute sinusitis. *Can Med Assoc J* 1997; **156**(6 Suppl): 1S–14S.

22 van Buchen FL, Knottnerus JA, Schrijnemaekers VJ, Peeters MF. Primary-care-based randomised placebo-controlled trial of antibiotic treatment in acute maxillary sinusitis. *Lancet* 1997; **349**: 683–7.

23 Del Mar CB, Glasziou PP. Antibiotics for the symptoms of sore throat (Cochrane Review). In: *The Cochrane Library,* Issue 1 1999. Oxford: Update Software, 1999.

24 Bracken M, Holford TR. Exposure to prescribed drugs in pregnancy and association with congenital malformations. *Obstet Gynecol* 1981; **58**: 336–44.

25 Saxen I. Epidemiology of cleft lip and palate: an attempt to rule out chance correlations. *Br J Prev Soc Med* 1975; **29**: 103–10.

26 Mangurten H H, Benawara R. Neonatal codeine withdrawal in infants of nonaddicted mothers. *Pediatrics* 1980; **65**: 159–60.

27 Dykes MHM. Evaluation of an antiasthmatic agent cromolyn sodium (Aarane, Intal). *JAMA* 1974; **227**: 1061–2.

28 Anonymous. Any place for depot triamcinolone in hay fever? *Drug Therapeut Bull* 1999; **37**(3): 17–18.

29. Schatz M, Pettiti D. Antihistamines and pregnancy. *Ann Allerg, Asthma and Immunol* 1997; **78**: 157–9.

30 Streissguth A P, Treder RP Barr HM *et al.* Aspirin and acetaminophen use by pregnant women and subsequent child IQ and attention decrements. *Teratology* 1987; **35**: 211–9.

31 Herz-Picciotto I, Hopenhayn-Rich C, Golub M *et al.* The risks and benefits of taking aspirin during pregnancy. *Epidemiol Rev* 1990; **12**: 108–48.

32 Reprorisk database. In: *Drugdex information system* (exp. 03/99). Denver, Colorado: Micromedex inc., 1999.

33 Stuart MJ Gross SJ Elrad H, Graeber JE. Effects of acetylsalicylic acid ingestion on maternal and neonatal haemostasis. *New Engl J Med* 1982; **307**: 902–12.

34 Lewis RN Schulman D. Influence of acetylsalicylic acid, an inhibitor of prostaglandin synthesis on the duration of human gestation and labour. *Lancet* 1973; **2**: 1159–61.

35 Norton ME, Merrill J, Cooper BAB, Kuller JA Clyman RI. Neonatal complications after the administration of indomethacin for preterm labour. *N Engl J Med* 1991; **329**: 1602–7.

36 Young GL Jewell MD. Topical treatment for vaginal candidiasis in pregnancy (Cochrane review). In: *The Cochrane Library*, Issue 4, 1998. Oxford: Update software, 1998.

37 Pursley T J Blomquist I K Abraham J Andersen H F, Bartley J A. Fluconazole-induced congenital anomalies in three infants. *Clin Infect Dis* 1996; **22**: 336–40.

38 Inman WH Pearce G, Wilton L. Safety of fluconazole in the treatment of vaginal candidiasis. A prescription-event monitoring study, with special reference to the outcome of pregnancy. *Eur J Clin Pharmacol* 1994; **46**: 115–8.

39 Mastriacovo P, Mazzone T, Botto LD *et al.* Prospective assessment of pregnancy outcomes after first trimester exposure to fluconazole. *Am J Obstet Gynecol* 1996; **9**: 1645–50.

40 Zeneca Pharma. Datasheet for Fulcin® (griseofulvin). In: *ABPI Compendium of data sheets and summaries of product characteristics 1998–9.* London: Datapharm Publications, 1998.

41 Novartis. Datasheet for Lamasil® (terbinafine). In: *ABPI Compendium of data sheets and summaries of product characteristics 1998–9.* London: Datapharm Publications, 1998.

42 Livingstone C. Lice and scabies. *Pharm J* 1998; **260**: 204–6.

43 Burgess I. Management guidelines for lice and scabies. *Prescriber* 1996; 7(9): 87–99.

44 Seton Healthcare. Datasheet for mebendazole (Pripsen) tablets. In: *ABPI Compendium of data sheets and summaries of product characteristics 1998–9.* London: Datapharm Publications, 1998.

45 Leach F. Management of threadworm infestation during pregnancy. *Arch Dis Childhood* 1990; **65**: 399–40.

3 Treatment and prevention of infection

TIMOTHY M A WELLER, RICHARD WISE

Key Points

- There is little evidence regarding the safety of most antimicrobial therapy in pregnancy.
- Clinical experience indicates the safety of penicillins and cephalosporins.
- Serious infections in pregnancy should be treated aggresively.

Introduction

Pregnant women are at the same risk of acquiring infectious diseases as anyone else, and are, indeed, more prone to some, such as urinary tract infections. It is, therefore, not uncommon for the use of antimicrobial agents to be considered during pregnancy. In some cases, including asymptomatic bacteriuria and bacterial vaginosis, therapy is primarily required to prevent fetal loss[1] or premature delivery[2] rather than for treatment of the mother. Whoever is the main beneficiary it is important to know which compounds can be used with negligible risk for minor infections and to have some appreciation of the balance of risks for more serious cases.

When risk to the fetus is being assessed, several points should be considered. With many antimicrobial agents, we now have more than 30 years' experience of freedom from congenital abnormality. Many studies have been performed in animals, the results of which, although important, should be viewed with some reservation. Sulphonamides, for example, can cause gross fetal malformations when given in high doses to rats and mice,[3] but teratogenicity has not been recorded in humans despite 50 years' use.

One of the reasons why laboratory animals make poor models for studying fetal damage is the profound effect antibiotics have on their normal gastrointestinal flora and consequently on the animal's metabolism. There are, however, some drugs with proven toxicity in humans which should definitely be avoided.

29

Streptomycin, for example, has caused neonatal ototoxicity after long-term treatment of maternal tuberculosis.[4,5] By implication the other aminoglycosides, gentamicin, tobramycin, netilmicin, and amikacin, should be avoided for minor infections, although there is no hard evidence that they have the same problem.

Changes in the dynamics of blood flow and other physiological effects of pregnancy can influence the pharmacokinetics of many drugs. Philipson showed that serum concentrations of ampicillin in women who were 9–36 weeks pregnant were half the values found in the same women when they were not pregnant.[6] Low maternal concentrations have been described after the ingestion of many antimicrobial agents, although the therapeutic implications of this are difficult to assess.

Failure of antibiotic treatment may be blamed incorrectly on the wrong choice of antibiotic, and the drug might be replaced by a potentially more toxic agent. This could be particularly dangerous when concern for the fetus prevents the doctor from giving high doses whilst treating a serious infection in the mother. In general, full adult doses should be used when treating infection in a pregnant woman. Similarly the length of therapy should be dictated by the disease and not be influenced unduly by the fact that the patient is pregnant. Inadequate treatment, which may be followed by further courses of antibiotics, is likely to put the mother and fetus at greater risk than a full course of the appropriate drug.

Antimicrobial agents

Table 3.1 lists most antimicrobial agents available in the UK together with their possible toxic effects on the fetus in early or late pregnancy. Each is given a safety rating:

- "Probably safe" indicates that no significant risk to the fetus has been documented and they are, therefore, a first choice drug if an antimicrobial agent has to be used.
- "Caution" indicates that effects on the fetus in animals have been recorded with the agent, or that its mode of action suggests a theoretical risk, or that there is insufficient data to be certain of its safety. There may, however, be times when the balance of risks suggests that such compounds should be used.
- "Avoid" indicates that the agent carries a definite risk and that it should only be used when there is a life-threatening condition for which no other drug is suitable.

Table 3.1 Antimicrobial agents and their possible adverse effects

Agent	Use	Adverse effects on fetus		Comments
		First trimester	Second and third trimester	
Penicillins				
penicillin V, penicillin G and long acting penicillins	Probably safe		Allergy; possibility of sensitizing the fetus	No adverse effects recorded during decades of use
ampicillin and amoxycillin	Probably safe		Allergy; possibility of sensitizing the fetus	No adverse effects recorded during decades of use
ampicillin pro-drugs (talampicillin, pivampicillin, bacampicillin)	Probably safe		Allergy; possibility of sensitizing the fetus	Limited data; no adverse effects recorded
co-amoxiclav (Augmentin)	Probably safe		Allergy; possibility of sensitizing the fetus	Limited data; no adverse effects recorded
ticarcillin, piperacillin and other antipseudomonal	Probably safe		Allergy; possibility of sensitizing the fetus	Limited data; no adverse effects recorded
flucloxacillin and other antistaphylococcal penicillins	Probably safe		Allergy; possibility of sensitizing the fetus	No adverse effects recorded during decades of use
Cephalosporins				
oral (cephalexin, cephradine, cefaclor, cefixime, cefpodoxime)	Probably safe		Allergy; possibility of sensitizing the fetus	Limited data; no adverse effects recorded
Intravenous (cefuroxime, cefotaxime, ceftazidime, ceftriaxone)	Probably safe		Allergy; possibility of sensitizing the fetus	Limited data; no adverse effects recorded

Table 3.1 *continued*

Agent	Use	Adverse effects on fetus		Comments
		First trimester	Second and third trimester	
Carbapenems imipenem/cilastatin (Primaxin)	Avoid			Toxicity in animals
meropenem	Caution			Limited data; use only if benefit outweighs risk
Macrolides/Lincosamides erythromycin base	Probably safe			No adverse effects recorded during decades of use
azithromycin, clarithromycin	Caution			Limited data; alternatives are usually available
clindamycin	Caution			Beware of maternal pseudomembranous colitis
Tetracyclines tetracycline, doxycycline, minocycline, oxytetracycline	Avoid	Effect on development in animals	Discoloration and dysplasia of bones and teeth, cataracts	Possible maternal hepatotoxicity
Aminoglycosides gentamicin, netilmicin, tobramycin, amikacin	Caution		Theoretical risk of ototoxicity	Use in serious sepsis if benefit outweighs risk
Quinolones ciprofloxacin, norfloxacin, ofloxacin, nalidixic acid	Avoid	Arthropathy in animal studies	Arthropathy in animal studies	May be used if no alternative available

Other antibacterial agents

chloramphenicol	Avoid	Grey baby syndrome	No evidence of ill effects to the fetus in early pregnancy but a safer agent is usually available
colistin	Avoid		Limited data; no adverse effects recorded
fosfomycin trometamol	Probably safe	Possible fetal toxicity	Limited data; no adverse effects recorded
fucidic acid	Probably safe		
metronidazole, tinidazole	Caution	Theoretical teratogenic risk	No adverse effects recorded; use if benefit outweighs risk
nitrofurantoin	Caution	Risk of haemolysis at term	Safe, except during labour and delivery
spectinomycin	Caution		Limited data; no adverse effects recorded
teicoplanin	Caution		Limited data; use only if benefit outweighs risk
trimethoprim	Avoid	Theoretical teratogenic risk	
co-trimoxazole (septrin)	Avoid	Theoretical teratogenic risk	
vancomycin	Caution	Neonatal haemolysis and methaemoglobinaemia	Limited data; no adverse effects recorded

continued overleaf

Table 3.1 *continued*

| Agent | Use | Adverse effects on fetus | | Comments |
		First trimester	Second and third trimester	
Antituberculous agents				
rifampicin	Caution	Teratogenic at high doses in animals	Possible increased risk of neonatal bleeding	Use only if benefit outweighs risk. Vitamin K should be given to mother and neonate. Avoid in mothers with liver disease
isoniazid	Probably safe			No adverse effects reported but teratogenic in animals
ethanmbutol	Caution	Teratogenic in animals		Limited data; use only when benefit outweighs risk
pyrazinamide	Caution			Safer agents always available
streptomycin	Avoid		Ototoxicity	
Antifungal agents				
amphotericin B	Caution			Limited data; use if benefit outweighs risk
fluconazole	Caution			Limited data; toxicity at high doses in animals; use only if benefit outweighs risk
itraconazole, ketoconazole	Avoid	Teratogenic in animals		Absorbed from vaginal topical use but no adverse effects recorded
miconazole, clotrimazole	Caution			
flucytosine	Avoid	Teratogenic in animals		Limited data, treatment may be postponed until after pregnancy
terbinafine	Caution			

griseofulvin	Avoid	Fetotoxic and teratogenic		Women should avoid pregnancy for 1 month following treatment
nystatin (topical)	Probably safe			Minimal absorption
Antimalarial agents				
chloroquine, hydroxychloroquine	Safe as prophylaxis			Safety has been established for low dose prophylaxis
quinine	Caution	Teratogenic in high doses	Ototoxicity occurs at high dose	Benefit may outweigh risk
primaquine	Avoid		Neonatal haemolysis and methaemoglobinaemia	Use only if unavoidable (see text)
mefloquine	Caution	Teratogenic in animals		Give folate supplements to the mother
proguanil	Probably safe			Use only if unavoidable (see text)
pyrimethamine and dapsone (Maloprim)	Caution	Theoretical teratogenic risk	Neonatal haemolysis and methaemoglobinaemia	
pyrimethamine and sulphadoxine (Fansidar)	Avoid	Theoretical teratogenic risk	Neonatal haemolysis and methaemoglobinaemia	
Antiparasitic agents				
albendazole, mebendazole, thiabendazole	Avoid	Teratogenic in animals		
piperazine	Probably safe			Limited data; treatment may be postponed until after pregnancy
praziquantel	Caution			Limited data; not on open market in UK

continued overleaf

Table 3.1 *continued*

Agent	Adverse effects on fetus			Comments
	Use	First trimester	Second and third trimester	
spiramycin	Probably safe			Limited data; not on open market in UK
pentamidine	Caution			Limited experience; use if benefit outweighs risk
Antiviral agents				
aciclovir, famciclovir, valaciclovir	Caution			Limited experience; use if benefit outweighs risk
ganciclovir	Avoid	Teratogenic in animals		
amantadine	Avoid	Embyrotoxic in animals		
vidarabine	Avoid	Teratogenic in animals		
foscarnet	Avoid			Manufacturer advises avoidance in pregnancy
Anti-HIV agents				
zidovudine	Probably safe			Treatment during pregnancy reduces risk of congenital infection
nucleoside analogues (didanosine, lamivudine, stavudine, zalcitabine)	Caution	Zalcitabine is teratogenic in animals		Limited data; use only if benefit outweighs risk
protease inhibitors (indinavir, ritonavir, saquinavir)	Caution			Limited data; use only if benefit outweighs risk

Treatment and prevention of specific infections

Table 3.2 lists some of the common infections likely to be encountered in pregnancy. The agents recommended are for empirical therapy and are, therefore, based on the pathogens most likely to cause each infection. Hence, it is particularly important to take cultures from pregnant patients *before* treatment so that a safe and efficacious change can be made if the patient does not respond or the causative organism proves resistant to initial therapy.

The first choice of treatment is usually an agent listed as "probably safe" in Table 3.1, although not necessarily so. A second choice may be used if the patient is allergic to the first compound or the bacteria responsible for the infection are resistant to it. Where one antibiotic is significantly better than all other therapies, it may be recommended, despite the need for caution when prescribing in pregnancy. Some of the conditions are not seen frequently enough in pregnancy for any suitable agent to be regarded as unequivocally safe. In such cases the problem has been highlighted in the Table, but specialist advice should be sought from an expert in the field before embarking on treatment. Finally, if an infection needs treating then it needs treating properly and, therefore, the dose chosen should be that which is normally used for the condition.

Prevention of infection in pregnancy protects both the mother and child. *Prophylaxis* should be given whenever the risk of disease outweighs the risk associated with the agent used to prevent it. Prophylactic regimens recommended in pregnancy are detailed in Table 3.3. In most cases they do not differ from those used for non-pregnant patients.

Urinary tract infection

The most common reason for a pregnant woman to take antibiotics is to treat acute cystitis or asymptomatic bacteriuria. The latter condition is associated with a significant incidence of pyelonephritis and possibly preterm delivery and low birthweight, making treatment essential.[1] It is recommended that antibiotics are administered for 7 days if bacteriuria is covert, but symptomatic infection usually responds to a shorter, 3–day, course.[7] In most cases amoxycillin (or its close relative, ampicillin) will be effective and safe. Where the causative organism is resistant (about one-third of urinary pathogens), an oral cephalosporin such as cephalexin or cephradine is suitable. Although the manufacturers

Table 3.2 Infections in pregnancy with recommended treatment

Condition	First choice treatment	Second choice treatment	Comments
Asymptomatic bacteriuria or simple cystitis	Ampicillin, amoxycillin, Co-amoxiclav or cephalexin by mouth	Nitrofurantoin (except at term) or fosfoymcin trometamol by mouth	7 days for asymptomatic bacteriuria, 3 days for cystitis
Acute pyelonephritis	Cefuroxime or co-amoxiclav intravenously		Treat for 7–10 days but may be oral when apyrexial for 24 hours
Pharyngitis	Phenoxymethylpenicillin by mouth or benzylpenicillin intravenously	Erythromycin	Antibiotics usually unnecessary as 70–80% caused by viruses
Sinusitis	Amoxycillin or co-amoxiclav		Antibiotics often unnecessary
Chest infection (mild)	Amoxycillin (+ erythromycin if atypicals suspected) by mouth	Erythromycin	As per British Thoracic Society recommendations[8]
Chest infection (severe)	Cefuroxime (+ erythromycin if atypicals suspected) intravenously		As per British Thoracic Society recommendations[8]
Tuberculosis	Rifampicin, isoniazid, pyrazinamide and ethambutol	Seek expert advice as many agents may be teratogenic	As per British Thoracic Society recommendations[9]
Skin/soft tissue/wound infection	Flucloxacillin	Clindamycin	
Bacterial vaginosis	Metronidazole	Co-amoxiclav	
Gonorrhoea	Penicillin	Cefotaxime or spectinomycin	
Chlamydia trachomatis	Erythromycin	Amoxycillin	
Pelvic inflammatory disease	Cefuroxime + erythromycin + metronidazole intravenously	Co-amoxiclav + erythromycin by mouth	
Listeriosis	Amoxycillin or ampicillin	Erythromycin	
Endocarditis: streptococcal staphylococcal	Benzylpenicillin + gentamicin Flucloxacillin		For full details see British Society for Antimicrobial Chemotherapy guidelines[18]
Meningitis	Benzylpenicillin	Cefotaxime	
Serious undiagnosed sepsis	Cefuroxime/cefotaxime ± gentamicin ± metronidazole		

Table 3.3 Antimicrobial prophlaxis in pregnancy

Condition	First choice prophylaxis	Second choice prophylaxis	Comments
Endocarditis	Amoxycillin	Clindamycin	As per British Society for Antimicrobial Chemotherapy guidelines[19]
Meningococcal meningitis	Rifampicin	Ceftriaxone intramuscularly	
Surgical prophylaxis			
clean surgery	No prophylaxis		
clean-contaminated surgery	Cefuroxime 1 dose		
contaminated surgery	Cefuroxime and metronidazole 1–3 doses		
Malaria	Chloroquine		See text for alternatives
Tuberculosis	Isoniazid		Give pyridoxine supplements with isoniazid

39

still recommend caution, co-amoxiclav does seem to be a safe alternative. Women who are allergic to beta-lactams can be given nitrofurantoin (except during labour or delivery) or fosfomycin trometamol.

There are occasions when *Pseudomonas aeruginosa* or other resistant isolates, insensitive to all the oral agents recommended above, are cultured. In these cases, it is important to establish that the organism is truly causing an infection, by repeating urine culture before treatment is undertaken. The patient may then have to be admitted to hospital for administration of a safe intravenous antibiotic, such as ceftazidime, or one that is potentially harmful, such as intramuscular gentamicin.

Lower respiratory tract infections

The most common bacterial pathogens of the lower respiratory tract, *Streptococcus pneumoniae* and *Haemophilus influenzae*, are usually sensitive to amoxycillin and ampicillin. These agents should, therefore, be the first choice for a mild community-acquired infection. A specimen should be taken for culture, however, as 10–15% of *H. influenzae* are resistant to these drugs. If this is the case, or the patient fails to respond, a course of co-amoxiclav may be indicated. Patients admitted to hospital with severe pulmonary infection should be treated with cefuroxime or cefotaxime according to the British Thoracic Society recommendations.[8]

Erythromycin has two indications in community-acquired lower respiratory tract infection:

- to treat pneumonia caused by "atypical" bacteria such as *Mycoplasma pneumoniae*, *Chlamydia pneumoniae* and *Legionella pneumophila*;
- for oral treatment of penicillin-allergic patients.

In both cases the newer macrolides, clarithromycin and azithromycin, are just as effective but they do not have the proven record of safety in pregnancy.

Tuberculosis

Although the possibility of teratogenesis was suspected with both rifampicin and ethambutol, they have been found to be safe in clinical practice. It is, therefore, recommended by the Joint Tuberculosis Committee of the British Thoracic Society that treatment of tuberculosis should be no different to that normally given.[9] Some caution is warranted in young women who use the oral contraceptive pill, as there is an increased risk of failure when rifampicin is prescribed. Of the second line agents, streptomycin is absolutely contraindicated in pregnancy because of the occurrence of ototoxicity in the fetus.[4,5] Ethionamide and prothionamide should only be used if no other compounds are available as they may be teratogenic.

Infections of the genital tract

Bacterial vaginosis has been associated with premature delivery[2] and treatment is, therefore, indicated if this condition is diagnosed during pregnancy. The antibiotic of choice, metronidazole, does have some theoretical risks but there have been no reports of problems in clinical use. Co-amoxiclav can be used as an alternative but is much less efficacious.

Gonorrhoea can be treated using a conventional course of penicillin in pregnancy. If the organism is resistant or the patient is allergic to penicillins, then spectinomycin is recommended. A third generation cephalosporins, such as cefotaxime or ceftriaxone, may be used instead.

Syphilis treatment in pregnancy does not differ from standard regimens. Therapy for the penicillin-allergic pregnant patient can be difficult because other agents, such as erythromycin, do not reliably treat the unborn child.[10] In such cases, expert advice should be sought as penicillin-desensitization of the patient may be the best option.

Chlamydia trachomatis infection during pregnancy should be treated with oral erythromycin. Patients unable to tolerate 500 mg four times a day for 7 days can be given 250 mg four times a day for 14 days. Alternatives are amoxycillin, which has a greater failure rate, or azithromycin, which has not been fully evaluated in pregnancy.

Pelvic inflammatory disease is not uncommon in pregnancy and treatment is difficult. Although many antibiotic combinations have been studied, inclusion of tetracycline is common and none specifically addresses therapy in pregnancy.[11] An acceptable intravenous regimen, based on the likely pathogens, would be cefuroxime (or cefotaxime) and erythromycin together with metronidazole. A less severe case can be treated with oral antibiotics such as a combination of co-amoxiclav and erythromycin.

Listeriosis

Infection with *Listeria monocytogenes* during pregnancy may result in spontaneous abortion, stillbirth, premature labour, or neonatal infection. Intravenous ampicillin or amoxycillin has been effective treatment for the mother and can prevent fetal damage. For patients allergic to penicillin, erythromycin is probably the best alternative.

Group B streptococcal colonization

Group B streptococci are normal inhabitants of the female genital tract and can cause neonatal meningitis and bacteraemia. Although this organism can often be detected throughout pregnancy, treatment of the mother prior to delivery is both ineffective and unnecessary. The use of intrapartum prophylaxis is controversial. Selective administration of ampicillin or benzylpenicillin to high risk patients has been shown to reduce the incidence of neonatal infection.[12] However, it still occurs in a small number of treated patients and also a significant number of those not selected. If prophylaxis is to be given during labour then intravenous ampicillin 2 g 8–hourly or benzylpenicillin 2.4 g 6–hourly until delivery is advised. Erythromycin can be used for penicillin-allergic women.

Serious sepsis

It is rare to have a pregnant patient with serious undiagnosed sepsis. When such a situation does occur, the risk to the mother outweighs any risk to the fetus. Therefore, the most appropriate antibiotics for the patients condition should be given in full doses. Once a pathogen and its antimicrobial susceptibilities have been identified, treatment can be directed at that organism. A suitable choice for empirical therapy would be a second or third generation cephalosporin (cefuroxime or cefotaxime), with the addition of gentamicin and/or metronidazole if this is warranted by the clinical condition. If an aminoglycoside is required, careful monitoring is needed to ensure that the patient is receiving sufficient drug, and that neither she nor the fetus is being exposed to unacceptably high levels.

Surgical prophylaxis

Although elective operations are avoided in pregnancy, emergency operations may be necessary. As in non-pregnant patients, a short course of an appropriate agent is indicated. If there is no evidence of established intra-abdominal sepsis, a parenteral cephalosporin such as cefuroxime plus metronidazole should be given. Alternatives include co-amoxiclav or clindamycin. The number of doses, one to three, depends upon the degree of contamination expected (see Table 3.3) and, if there is proven infection at operation, then 3–5 days treatment is required.

The risk of infection following emergency caesarean section is substantial and the need for prophylactic antibiotics is clear. There is a smaller risk after an elective procedure but most practitioners still give peri-operative antibiotics. One dose of cefuroxime, with or without metronidazole, ought to be sufficient provided it is given early enough to be present in the tissues when the incision is made. Thus, it should be administered before or during induction of anaesthesia. There is no advantage, and in fact it is a significant disadvantage, in delaying prophylaxis until after the cord has been clamped.

Malaria prophylaxis and treatment

Malaria is an important cause of abortion, premature labour, and perinatal death, and it affects the mother as well. Pregnant women should be advised strongly against visiting endemic areas, especially those where chloroquine resistance exists. If a visit to an area of malaria transmission is unavoidable, then prophylaxis is indicated during pregnancy. It should be started 1 week before a malarial zone is visited and continued for 1 month after leaving. For travel to places where resistance is not a problem, chloroquine 300 mg weekly is recommended. This can be combined with proguanil 200 mg daily which also has a good record of safety in pregnancy. Travel to a country where chloroquine-resistant *Plasmodium falciparum* is encountered, presents a problem as there are doubts about all other effective agents. It is suggested that mefloquine or sulphone/diaminopyrimidine (Maloprim), supplemented with folic acid, can be used with caution and, if it is taken inadvertently in the first trimester, this is not an indication for termination.[13] However, even these do not give complete protection where parasites are multidrug resistant and complete avoidance of danger areas is preferable.

Chloroquine can be used to treat malaria caused by *P. vivax, P. ovale* and *P. malariae* and also *P. falciparum* from areas where resistance is not a problem. Although quinine is reported to be teratogenic in guineapigs, few adverse effects have been recorded in pregnant women despite widespread use, and this remains the treatment of choice.

Toxoplasmosis

A diagnosis of acute toxoplasmosis can be established in the mother by detection of specific IgM or a rise in maternal IgG. Fetal

43

infection can only be confirmed by the isolation of parasites from fetal blood. It is relatively uncommon in the first trimester, but in most of the cases that do occur the disease is severe. In the third trimester, however, infection of the fetus is more usual, but most babies will have no overt disease at birth.

Management of toxoplasmosis in pregnancy requires specialist knowledge and liaison with an expert is advised. Maternal infection can be treated using spiramycin 3 g/day in three to four divided doses for 3 weeks, but the amount of drug crossing the placenta is not sufficient to treat the fetus. Therefore, if there is fetal infection, the mother should also receive pyrimethamine 25 mg/day and sulphadiazine 4 g/day with folic acid supplements for the same 3 weeks.[14] This regimen is followed by spiramycin 3 g/day for 3 weeks, alternating with no treatment for the same period until term.

Vaccination

As a general rule immunization during pregnancy should be avoided if possible, although most vaccines are probably safe to give. Particular caution is advised in relation to the live vaccines.[15] Immunization against rubella is contraindicated during pregnancy and conception should be avoided in the month following administration of the vaccine. Similarly, polio vaccine should not be given in the first 4 months of pregnancy. In circumstances when there is a significant risk of disease, following exposure to hepatitis B positive blood or travel to an area endemic for yellow fever for instance, then the benefit gained by immunization of the mother may well outweigh the risk to the fetus.

HIV

It has been shown that the rate of HIV transmission from mother to child is significantly reduced if zidovudine is used during pregnancy.[16] Prophylaxis is, therefore, currently recommended for all HIV-infected pregnant women to prevent vertical transmission.[17] Other antiretroviral drugs are relatively new, and little experience has been gained of their use in pregnancy. As more information on the efficacy and safety of these agents becomes available in the future, a combination regimen may be found to be more effective. Even without these data, it is recommended that women currently receiving therapy for HIV infection should remain on the same drugs throughout pregnancy.[17]

Table 3.4   Antibiotics to be used with caution or avoided whilst breast feeding

Agent	Use	Comments
Amantadine	Avoid	Toxicity has been reported in infants
Chloramphenicol	Avoid	Possibility of infant marrow suppression
Ganciclovir	Avoid	Adverse effects in animal studies; avoid breast feeding until 72 hours after last dose
Isoniazid	Caution	Theoretical risk of convulsions or neuropathy; both mother and baby should receive pyridoxine supplements
Metronidazole	Caution	Theoretical risk of mutagenesis; gives breast milk an unpleasant taste.
Nitrofurantoin	Caution	Small risk of haemolysis in glucose-6-phosphate dehydrogenase-deficient infants
Quinolones	Avoid	High concentrations in breast milk; may affect cartilage development in weight-bearing joints
Sulphonamides (including co-trimoxazole)	Caution	Small risk of kernicterus in jaundiced infants; haemolysis in glucose-6-phosphate dehydrogenase-deficient infants
Tetracyclines	Avoid	Chelation of tetracycline by calcium ions in milk probably prevents risk of teeth discoloration but still not recommended

Antibiotics and lactation

Both mother and general practitioner are often anxious that antimicrobial agents being used to treat the mother are being transferred to the infant. Although most antibiotics are found in breast milk in low concentrations, they are unlikely to affect the child. This is because either the agent will not be absorbed from the child's gastrointestinal tract in appreciable amounts or the concentrations reached in the infant are extremely low. Table 3.4 gives details of the few antimicrobials that should be used with caution or avoided during breastfeeding.

References

1   Condie AP, Brumfitt W, Reeves DS, Williams JD. The effects of bacteriuria in pregnancy on foetal health. In: Brumfitt W, Asscher AW, eds. *Urinary tract infection*. London: Oxford University Press, 1973.
2   Krohn MA, Hillier SL, Lee ML, Rabe LK, Eschenbach DA. Vaginal Bacteroides species are associated with an increased rate of preterm delivery among women in preterm labor. *J Infect Dis* 1991; **164**: 88–93.
3   Kato T, Kitagawa S. Production of congenital abnormalities in the fetuses of rats and mice with various sulphonamides. *Congen Abnormal* 1973; **13**: 7–15.

4 Assael BM, Parini R, Rusconi F. Ototoxicity of aminoglycoside antibiotics in infants and children. *Pediatr Infect Dis* 1982; **1**: 357–67.

5 Conway N, Birt BD. Streptomycin in pregnancy: effect on the foetal ear. *BMJ* 1966; ii: 260–3.

6 Philipson A. Pharmacokinetics of antibiotics in pregnancy and labour. *Clin Pharmacokinet* 1979; **4**: 297–309.

7 Bint AJ, Hill D. Bacteriuria in pregnancy – an update on significance, diagnosis and management. *J Antimicrob Chemother* 1994; **33** (Suppl. A): 93–7.

8 The British Thoracic Society. Guidelines for the management of community-acquired pneumonia in adults admitted to hospital. *Br J Hosp Med* 1993; **49**: 346–50.

9 Ormerod LP. Chemotherapy and management of tuberculosis in the United Kingdom: recommendations of the Joint Tuberculosis Committee of the British Thoracic Society. *Thorax* 1990; **45**: 403–8.

10 Hashisaki P, Wertzberger GG, Conrand GL, Nichols CR. Erythromycin failure in the treatment of syphilis in pregnant women. *Sex Transm Dis* 1983; **10**: 36–8.

11 Peterson HB, Walker CK, Kahn JG, Washington AE, Eschenbach DA, Faro S. Pelvic inflammatory disease. Key treatment issues and options. *JAMA* 1991; **266**: 2605–11.

12 Omenaca Teres F, Matorras R, Garcia Perea A, Elorza MD. Prevention of neonatal group B streptococcal sepsis. *Pediatr Infect Dis J* 1987; **6**: 874.

13 Bradley DJ, Warhurst DC. Guidelines for the prevention of malaria in travellers from the United Kingdom. *CDR Review* 1997; **7**: R137–51.

14 Wong S-Y, Remington JS. Toxoplasmosis in pregnancy. *Clin Infect Dis* 1994; **18**: 853–62.

15 Salisbury DM, Begg NT, eds. *Immunisation against infectious disease*. London: HMSO, 1996.

16 Connor EM, Sperling RS, Gelber R *et al*. Reduction of maternal-infant transmission of human immunodeficiency virus type 1 with zidovudine treatment. *New Engl J Med* 1994; **331**: 1173–80.

17 Minkoff H, Augenbraun M. Antiretroviral therapy for pregnant women. *Am J Obstet Gynecol* 1997; **176**: 478–89.

18 Working Party of the British Society for Antimicrobial Chemotherapy. Antibiotic treatment of streptococcal, enterococcal, and staphylococcal endocarditis. *Heart* 1998; **79**: 207–10.

19 Simmons NA. Recommendations for endocarditis prophylaxis. *J Antimicrob Chemother* 1993; **31**: 437–8.

4 Anticoagulants

MICHAEL DE SWIET

Key points

- Women at high risk of thromboembolism should receive subcutaneous LMWH throughout pregnancy.

- Lower risk women should be given aspirin antenatally, with heparin during labour and for 6 weeks postnatally.

- Thromboprophylaxis should be considered at delivery for patients who:

    - have had bed rest for at least a week

    - are obese

    - are over 35

    - are in their fourth or greater pregnancy

    - are having a caesarean section.

Introduction

Anticoagulant therapy is used in pregnancy to prevent and treat potentially life-threatening disasters such as pulmonary embolus, cerebral embolus, and thrombosis of artificial heart valves; indeed pulmonary embolus (with hypertension) is the leading cause of maternal mortality in the United Kingdom.[1] However, used incorrectly, anticoagulants have the potential to cause equally serious bleeding in the mother and fetus, and long-term heparin treatment can also cause bone demineralization. So the proper use of anticoagulants is a crucial part of modern obstetric practice. This chapter considers the use of anticoagulants in both venous thromboembolic disease and in patients with heart disease who are at risk of systemic thromboembolism.

Heparin and low molecular weight heparin

Heparin is an acid mucopolysaccharide with varying chain lengths of molecular weight between 4000 and 40 000 Daltons. Heparin has some thrombolytic action but, in general, it is used to prevent further blood clotting rather than lyse clots that are already present. The higher molecular weight heparins also inhibit platelet activity.

The heterogeneous chain length preparations of heparin have been fractionated into those of low molecular weight (LMWH). LMWH is used quite extensively for thromboprophylaxis in high risk surgery outside pregnancy, e.g. in orthopaedic patients or in cancer patients. Several different LMWHs are available from different manufacturers, e.g. certoparin, dalteparin, enoxaparin, tinzaparin. Their effects are similar, though not necessarily identical in view of the different ways in which each manufacturer has fractionated the heparin molecules. Studies in pregnancy have been reported with enoxaparin[2-5] and dalteparin.[6,7] LMWH has a relatively greater anti-Xa effect than antithrombin effect. This, together with the lack of antiplatelet activity, may decrease the risk of bleeding with the use of LMWH while maintaining antithrombotic activity.[8] From the patients' point of view, a major advantage is that, for thromboprophylaxis, LMWH only needs to be given once rather than twice daily as is the practice with unfractionated heparin. Also the injections tend to be less painful.[9] At present increased cost is the major disadvantage. Depending on local purchasing agreements, LMWH can cost between three and seven times as much as unfractionated heparin.[10,11]

Because of their high polarity and lack of lipid solubility none of the forms of heparin cross the placenta.[6,12] Also none is excreted in breast milk. Heparin-induced thrombocytopenia (HIT) is a possible and serious complication of all forms of heparin treatment.[13] Thrombocytopenia either presents acutely as a result of platelet aggregation or occurs 7–10 days after treatment starts, because of an interaction between platelets, heparin, and a specific IgG autoantibody.[14,15] HIT may cause bleeding,[16] but paradoxically further clotting is a more common consequence.[14,17] HIT is very rare in women in the reproductive age group and probably even rarer in patients taking LMWH[18-20] than in those taking unfractionated heparin. In pregnancy LMWH has been shown to cause less platelet aggregation than does unfractionated heparin.[21] HIT reoccurs if patients are re-exposed to heparin. About 40% of patients who get HIT with unfractionated heparin will also get it on treatment with LMWH.

Orgaron

In a patient who has had HIT, the heparinoid orgaron may be used as an alternative, although about 10% of such patients will also get HIT with orgaron. There are anecdotal reports of the use of orgaron in pregnancy.[22] It appears not to cross the placenta. By comparison with any form of heparin it is very expensive.

Warfarin

Warfarin is a form of coumarin that antagonizes Vitamin K. In general warfarin is confined to long-term anticoagulation rather than acute management, and in pregnancy there is the additional problem that the drug crosses the placenta and can therefore affect the fetus. However, warfarin is not excreted in breast milk. Numerous other drugs, and even avocado pears,[23] interact with warfarin and can dangerously potentiate or reduce its effect.

Thrombolytic drugs

These drugs lyse clots by activating plasminogen to produce plasmin which breaks down the cross links of fibrin within the thrombus. First generation agents streptokinase and urokinase have had limited use in pregnancy. Newer and more fibrin specific agents, such as alteplase and anistreplase, have not been evaluated in pregnancy. Bleeding is the major complication. There is no evidence that there is less risk with the newer drugs.

Deep vein thrombosis and pulmonary embolism

After emergency resuscitation for pulmonary embolus, the treatment of both deep vein thrombosis and pulmonary embolus may be divided into an initial acute phase, which lasts for up to a week, and a subsequent chronic phase lasting for several months. In the chronic phase, in particular, the aim of therapy is to prevent further incidents of thromboembolism.

Acute phase treatment

Heparin

Most cases of venous thromboembolism are treated initially with heparin. To prevent further clot formation, relatively high blood levels of heparin must be achieved. Although up to 40 000 units of heparin per day have been given subcutaneously, this is not usually practical because of bruising and irregular absorption. The initial treatment should be with intravenous heparin: a 5000 unit bolus is given first followed by 40 000 units per day (approximately 1600 units per hour) by continuous infusion. The aim is to achieve a level of 0.6–1.0 unit per ml (as assayed by the protamine sulphate neutralization test) or to double the APTT when compared to control. Heparin is not stable in dextrose and should therefore be given in saline, preferably made up in a small volume of 10–20 ml and very slowly infused with a constant infusion pump. Apart from HIT (see above), the only side effect of acute heparin administration is bleeding, although its preservative, chlorbutol, may cause hypotension[24] (side effects of prolonged therapy are considered below).

If it is necessary to reverse heparin therapy; merely stopping the infusion will be sufficient for most patients given intravenous heparin. There will be undetectable levels in the blood 6 hours after therapy has stopped. If the situation is more urgent, the patient can be given protamine 1 mg per 100 units of administered heparin. When a continuous infusion of heparin is being given, twice the quantity of protamine should be given to neutralize the hourly dose. No more than 50 mg of protamine should be given in a 10–minute period, since protamine itself can cause bleeding. Protamine can also be used to reverse LMWH, but there is very little experience of its use in these circumstances.

Initial phase, high dose intravenous heparin therapy is continued for an arbitrary period of 3–7 days; the length of treatment depends on the severity of the initial episode of venous thromboembolism and whether there is any evidence of recurrence. Studies of intravenous heparin given for only 5 days[25] have not been performed in pregnancy, and have only been performed in the non-pregnant state in patients with deep vein thrombosis, not pulmonary embolus.

Promising studies have been reported in non-pregnant patients using fixed dose subcutaneous low molecular weight heparin (logiparin,[26] fraxiparin[27]) in the initial phase of treatment. In the study of Hull,[26] not only were there the obvious advantages of subcutaneous fixed dose versus adjusted dose intravenous therapy, but there was less bleeding in the acute phase and fewer recurrences.

In pregnancy there is more experience with enoxaparin, particularly for thromboprophylaxis,[2] but a recent anecdotal report describes the use of adjusted dose subcutaneous enoxaparin 1 mg/kg bodyweight given twice daily for acute treatment of thromboembolism in pregnancy.[5] These high doses were continued through pregnancy though the dose was reduced to 40 mg every 12 hours during delivery. Such treatment could be a real advance in the management of deep vein thrombosis and pulmonary embolus in pregnancy: a twice daily, subcutaneous regimen that might eventually be fixed dose without the need for hematological monitoring would be much easier to use than intravenous therapy with the dose adjusted according to the APTT. However, we cannot extrapolate directly from the trials in non-pregnant patients since they were of subcutaneous LMWH compared to unfractionated intravenous heparin, with both backed up by treatment with warfarin beginning at the same time or soon after the initiation of heparin therapy.

In pregnancy, warfarin would not be used and therefore the patient is dependent solely on the anticoagulant effect of subcutaneous LMWH. This may indeed be sufficient, providing the dose requirements are the same in pregnancy as in the non-pregnant state. However, until more experience is gained, high dose subcutaneous LMWH cannot be recommended for standard treatment of thromboembolism in pregnancy.

The alternatives to heparin in the initial phase of treatment are surgery, catheter fragmentation and thrombolytic therapy. All these alternatives have the advantage of therapy directed towards removing or breaking up the initial clot. All should be considered in the pregnant and non-pregnant states for initial treatment in patients with major pulmonary embolus or massive iliofemoral deep vein thrombosis, although surgery and catheter fragmentation are outside the scope of this chapter. (So too is the use of caval filters for prevention of recurrent pulmonary embolism.)

Thrombolysis

Pfeiffer[28] claimed successful treatment of deep vein thrombosis in 12 pregnant patients given streptokinase as a loading dose (250 000 units by intravenous infusion over 20 minutes) followed by an infusion of 160 000 units per hour for 4 hours, with subsequent alteration of the infusion rate depending on the plasma thrombin time. Bell and Meek[28] discount the necessity for adjusting the dosage schedule and would recommend a maintenance therapy of 100 000 iu per hour for 24–72 hours after the initial loading dose. Although Pfeiffer[30] suggests that very little streptokinase crosses the human placenta, pregnancy is considered a minor contraindication to the use of thrombolytic therapy; subsequent delivery within 10 days is a major contraindication to thrombolytic therapy.[31] Since it is possible that thrombolytic therapy may precipitate premature labour by causing an increase in circulating plasminogen levels,[32] there is a risk that the relatively minor contraindication will become a major contraindication. However, it has also been suggested that streptokinase therapy will cause relative uterine atony because of the interference of fibrin degradation products with uterine contraction.[33]

If it is necessary to reverse thrombolytic therapy in pregnancy, aprotinin, which has large molecules and does not cross the placenta, should be used rather than aminocaproic acid. However, apart from the 12 patients treated in pregnancy by Pfeiffer,[28] other studies are only case reports,[32,34] and therefore there is really still not sufficient experience to recommend the use of thrombolytic agents in pregnancy except in exceptional circumstances,[35] such as life-threatening pulmonary embolus. In our experience, streptokinase appeared to be life saving in a patient who was moribund from pulmonary embolus in pregnancy – but the cost was severe bleeding from a normally sited placenta.

Chronic phase treatment

Warfarin

It is established that there is a definite, though low, incidence of teratogenesis associated with the use of warfarin in the first trimester of pregnancy.[36-39] The most common syndrome is chondrodysplasia punctata, in which cartilage and bone formation is abnormal.[37-40] The asplenia syndrome[41] and diaphragmatic herniae have also been reported.[42] It has also been recognized that the use of warfarin in late pregnancy after 36 weeks' gestation is associated with serious retroplacental and intracerebral fetal bleeding,[43] since warfarin does cross the placenta, unlike heparin. However, the question has arisen as to whether oral anticoagulants should be used at all in pregnancy,[44] even after the first trimester, because of the risk of fetal malformation. It has been suggested that warfarin causes repeated small intracerebral haemorrhages and that these are the causes of the optic atrophy, microcephaly, and mental retardation.[45] Gross subdural haemorrhage may also occur in the fetus before 36 weeks gestation.[46]

The teratogenic risks may not be so great as anecdotal reports would suggest. Chen et al.[47] studied the outcome of 22 pregnancies, where the mother had taken warfarin in the first trimester, and 20 pregnancies where warfarin had been taken between 13 and 36 weeks. Warfarin was being used in the management of artificial heart valves. Although the spontaneous abortion rate was high (36% in those taking warfarin), there were no cases of chondrodysplasia punctata or microcephaly. We compared the infants of 20 patients who had taken warfarin in the second and third trimesters with those of well-matched controls, and found no difference in intellectual attainment at a mean age of 4 years.[48] Microcephaly is therefore unlikely to be common in the children of women taking warfarin. It may relate to the method of monitoring used for warfarin therapy and therefore to the amount of warfarin taken. CNS malformations do seem more common in those taking higher doses of warfarin. The high abortion rate found in the study by Chen et al.[47] is probably real, and an increased risk of abortion should therefore be considered another fetal complication of warfarin therapy.

For the mother, bleeding also appears to be more of a problem in patients treated with warfarin than in those treated with heparin, even if the patients have prothrombin times within the normal therapeutic range.[49] Fetomaternal haemorrhage has also been reported.[50]

For all the above reasons conventional warfarin therapy should not be used in the chronic phase of treatment of venous thromboembolism in pregnancy, or in the first week of the puerperium. The only situation where warfarin therapy is recommended in pregnancy is in the management of some patients with artificial heart valves or mitral valve disease (see below). Patients may continue to breastfeed,[51] since there is no detectable secretion of warfarin in breast milk.[52] This is not so for phenindione where maternal therapy has caused severe haemorrhage in a breastfed infant.[53] However, phenindione may not be so teratogenic as warfarin;[54] unfortunately, there are not sufficient data to confirm this suggestion.

Heparin

Subcutaneous, self-administered heparin is the preferred chronic phase treatment for venous thromboembolism in pregnancy,[55] since it does not have the risks of warfarin. (The possible complications of long-term heparin therapy are described below in the section on Thromboprophylaxis).

The majority of patients are given acute phase high dose intravenous heparin therapy for 7–10 days, although some with massive deep vein thrombosis or severe pulmonary embolus may benefit from intravenous heparin for up to 14 days. The patients are then given subcutaneous heparin. Any form of heparin may be used subcutaneously in the chronic phase of treatment, although the tendency is increasingly towards LMWH. If unfractionated heparin is chosen, give 10 000 units subcutaneously twice daily and check the anti-Xa heparin level about 4 hours after dosing. Provided there is detectable heparin activity, it is not usual to increase the dose of heparin above 10 000 units every 12 hours. If the heparin assay exceeds 0.2 units per millilitre, the dose is reduced, since such levels are associated with excessive bleeding.[56] Heparin levels are stable in patients who are taking subcutaneous heparin, but because of pregnancy-induced changes in blood volume and renal handling of heparin, and because treatment with heparin may continue for up to six months, repeated heparin assays should be made, about as frequently as the patient attends for normal antenatal visits.

The anti-Xa heparin assay with the currently available kits has become easier to perform and more widely available. However, an acceptable alternative is to measure the thrombin time which is even more widely available as part of the normal clotting screen. The thrombin time is very sensitive to heparin, and patients who are taking more than prophylactic levels of heparin show a marked prolongation of the thrombin time. Therefore the risk of bleeding in patients taking subcutaneous heparin can be assessed with the thrombin time: if it is not prolonged, the patients are unlikely to bleed because of heparin treatment.

If a single daily injection of LMWH is to be given, recommended doses are enoxaparine 40 mg, dalteparin 5000 units, or tinzaparin 50 units /kg. Although treatment with LMWH does not require monitoring in the non-pregnant state, the safety of this approach has not been established in pregnancy. At present it is recommended that the anti-Xa level and/or thrombin and APTT times are checked as described above for unfractionated heparin treatment. However, LMWH is less likely to affect the APTT and thrombin times than is unfractionated heparin. So if there is real concern about the risk of bleeding, anti-Xa levels should be performed.

The relative advantages of LMWH compared to unfractionated heparin have been considered above. However, the Author favours LMWH in the chronic phase of thromboembolism treatment, because of once daily administration, and the possible superior profile of antithrombotic effect compared to bleeding risk, despite the increased cost. Also in terms of anti-Xa activity, subcutaneous enoxaparin given 40 mg once daily to puerperal women has a more favourable profile than does unfractionated heparin in the recommended post-partum dose of 7500 units twice daily.[10]

Because of the high incidence of thromboembolism in the days following labour and delivery,[1] subcutaneous heparin administration should be continued through labour. The heparin assay or thrombin time can be checked in the week preceding delivery, since patients attend the hospital weekly at this time in pregnancy. There is no increased risk of intra- or post-partum haemorrhage in these patients,[4,57,58] although those who inadvertently take too much heparin are at risk of bleeding.[59] Provided that the thrombin time is normal, it is now believed that epidural block is not contraindicated.[60] The risk of epidural haematoma[61,62] is very small.[62]

At delivery, the dose of unfractionated subcutaneous heparin is empirically reduced to 7500 units b.d. because of the contraction in circulating blood volume and because the clotting factors return to normal levels during the puerperium. However, the dose of LMWH does not need to be altered because of its bioavailability is more consistent and there is a probable lower risk of bleeding for a given level of thromboprophylaxis. The heparin assay is checked at least once after delivery, if the patient continues to take subcutaneous heparin for the recommended 6 weeks post partum. Alternatively, 1 week after delivery, when the risk of secondary post-partum haemorrhage is much less, the patient may take warfarin rather than heparin. In either case breastfeeding is safe. Heparin is not secreted in breast milk and would not be absorbed from the infant's stomach. Warfarin is not excreted in breast milk.[52] The option as to whether to continue heparin or to switch to warfarin depends on which the patient finds less inconvenient.

Therapy with heparin initiated in pregnancy, or warfarin if introduced after 7 days post partum, is continued for an arbitrary period of 6 weeks post partum, at which time the extra risk of thromboembolism associated with pregnancy is considered to have passed. Patients who develop venous thromboembolism in the puerperium should be treated as above, except that, after the acute phase, warfarin may be used alone in chronic phase treatment if it is not given for the first 7 days after delivery. The total length of anticoagulant treatment should be at least 3 months.

Prophylaxis of thromboembolism

There are two groups of patients in whom prophylaxis might be considered: those who are at high risk because of age, parity, obesity, or operative delivery,[1] and those who have had thromboembolism in the past.[63] With regard to the former group, it is generally believed (although not proven) that the risk of thromboembolism is greatest in the puerperium and therefore that any prophylaxis need only be used during this period and to cover labour. The Confidential Maternal Mortality Series[64] very clearly shows that the risks of thromboembolism are increased markedly with increasing age. If these and other data are applied, there is a case for using some form of prophylaxis such as low dose heparin in all patients who have had bed rest for at least 1 week before delivery, the obese, and also in those over the age of 35 or in their fourth pregnancy (excluding abortion), even if they have a spontaneous vaginal delivery.[65] The Royal College of Obstetricians and Gynaecologists of the United Kingdom has also drawn up guidelines for thromboprophylaxis in those being delivered by caesarean section.[66] None of the above recommendations has been evaluated by clinical trial.

The second group of patients are those who have had thromboembolism in the past; they are considered to be at risk throughout pregnancy. Warfarin prophylaxis seems unacceptable because of the maternal and fetal complications of warfarin therapy outlined above. Dextran should no longer be used for thromboprophylaxis in pregnancy; there had always been concern about the risk of anaphylactic reactions, but it is now realized that in pregnancy such reactions may be accompanied by severe uterine hypertonus; in turn these reactions have caused fetal hypoxia with subsequent brain damage.

The alternative is to use subcutaneous heparin throughout pregnancy. However, since these patients are asymptomatic at the beginning of treatment and because the treatment is only being used prophylactically, the safety of such therapy for mother and fetus must be established even more rigorously than in the treatment of established venous thromboembolism.

Heparin

The most obvious maternal complication is bruising at the injection site. This can be reduced by good injection technique but rarely eliminated. Although this is undoubtedly an inconvenience, and at times painful, most mothers tolerate a degree of bruising. A further maternal complication of prolonged heparin therapy is osteoporosis (heparin-induced ostopenia).[67-69] Griffith *et al.*[70] reported that heparin-induced osteopenia only occurs in patients receiving more than 15 000 units of heparin per day for at least 6 months; but bone demineralization has been reported following the administration of only 10 000 units of heparin per day in pregnancy for 19 weeks.[71] Based on one series of 184 women receiving heparin thromboprophylaxis in pregnancy, the risk of symptomatic fractures is about 2%.[72] The cause of the osteopenia is unknown. Since heparin-induced osteopenia is much more common in pregnancy, it is likely that the enhanced bone turnover of pregnancy[73] and the fetal demand for calcium[74] are contributing factors. A follow-up study of those patients who are taking subcutaneous heparin suggests that even those patients who are asymptomatic may have some degree of bone demineralization.[74] This is particularly worrying because of fears that the osteoporosis will progress further at the menopause. Fortunately a follow-up study from Sweden based on radiological assessment of the spine suggests that heparin-induced osteopenia does regress once heparin treatment has been stopped.[75] Also, Ginsberg *et al.*[76] studied 61 patients, 2 years after stopping long-term heparin treatment, and found no difference in bone density when they were compared with controls. Both of these studies suggest that heparin-induced osteoporosis regresses on cessation of therapy.

Occasionally heparin causes alopecia and allergic reactions including skin necrosis.[77] Allergic reactions are usually local and seem to be more common with subcutaneous than intravenous therapy. Indeed very cautious intravenous therapy with added hydrocortisone has been used in a patient allergic to subcutaneous therapy.[78] In patients who are allergic to one form of heparin given subcutaneously, it is worth trying other heparin or LMWH preparations. However, in these circumstances most patients are allergic to all types of heparin that are tried.

In one study of non-pregnant patients, fraxiparin was shown to cause modest rises in the serum potassium.[79] It is not known whether this is specific to fraxiparin. In a single pregnant patient enoxaparin has been shown to cause severe hyperlipidaemia.[22] Heparin may cause thrombocytopenia as noted above.

Because of the maternal complications of prolonged subcutaneous heparin therapy, heparin should not be used indiscriminately for prophylaxis throughout pregnancy in all patients who have had thromboembolism in the past. Our present approach[4,80,81] is to counsel patients about the relative risks of prophylactic therapy and recurrence of thromboembolism in the antenatal period. Subcutaneous heparin is only used throughout pregnancy in those patients who are considered particularly at risk, having had thromboembolism more than once in the past, or having acquired or inherited abnormalities of the clotting or thrombolytic systems and a single episode of thromboembolism in the past. Acquired abnormalities that may complicate pregnancy are the presence of lupus anticoagulant and/or anticardiolipin antibodies (antiphospholipid syndrome). Inherited abnormalities of current concern are antithrombin III, protein C and S deficiencies, factor V Leiden, prothrombin gene mutation, hyperhomocystinaemia, and homocsytinuria. Patients are also considered at high risk if they have had an episode of thromboembolism and a family history of thromboembolism in a first-degree relative suggesting that they have an undetected form of inherited thrombophilia.

Subcutaneous heparin is also used in those patients who themselves are particularly concerned about the risk of repeated thromboembolism. In addition, we use subcutaneous heparin in low risk patients who have only had a single episode of thromboembolism at times when they are most at risk, such as during admission to hospital for surgery or bed rest. High risk patients take heparin starting when they book for pregnancy care. The heparin is given as described above regarding chronic phase therapy for the management of established thromboembolism in pregnancy. They are monitored haematologically in the same way. After delivery the patients receive subcutaneous heparin for at least 1 week, and either subcutaneous heparin or warfarin for a further 5 weeks making a total of 6 weeks' postnatal treatment. Again the Author favours the use of LMWH rather than unfractionated heparin for the same reasons as given above. The choice between warfarin and heparin after delivery again depends on which treatment the patient finds less inconvenient (see above). As in the treatment of an established case of thromboembolism in pregnancy (see above), the length of time for which prophylaxis is continued after delivery is 6 weeks, although this is arbitrary.

Patients who have only had a single episode of thromboembolism in the past, no matter what the associated circumstances, are considered at low risk of recurrence in pregnancy. These patients start taking aspirin 75 mg once daily at booking and then enter the above schedule when they present in labour or at elective delivery. They are given LMWH or unfractionated heparin and are then managed in the same way as the high risk patients. The justification for the use of aspirin is that meta-analysis indicates that antiplatelet drugs reduce the risk of deep vein thrombosis and pulmonary embolus by 36% to 60% ,[82] although no trials of low dose aspirin have been performed in pregnancy for thromboprophylaxis. Nevertheless, there have been extensive trials of low dose aspirin for the prevention of pre-eclampsia.[83] Although the efficacy of aspirin for this indication is questionable, the safety record for both mother and fetus is good.

Although the regimen for low risk patients is a compromise since it does not provide any cover during the antenatal period before labour, we have not observed any cases of antenatal or postnatal thromboembolism in 47 pregnancies treated in Queen Charlotte's Hospital in this way.[84] All the patients had been treated for at least 6 weeks for an episode of deep vein thrombosis or pulmonary embolism before the index pregnancy. In 47% of patients the previous episode had occurred in pregnancy, in 33% it had occurred when the patient was taking the Pill. It therefore seems likely that the study of Badaraco and Vessey,[63] which suggests a 12% risk of thromboembolism in patients who have had deep vein thrombosis or pulmonary embolism in the past, very much overestimates the risk of antenatal thromboembolism; the risk appears to be of the order of 2% or less.

Anticoagulant therapy for patients with heart disease

This is a major problem in the management of patients with heart disease in pregnancy. Anticoagulant therapy is most frequently necessary in patients with artificial valve replacements, but it may also be used in those with atrial fibrillation and those who have pulmonary hypertension owing to pulmonary vascular disease. At present the anticoagulant of choice is warfarin which should be used until about 37 weeks' gestation, even though the risk of fetal malformation such as optic atrophy may persist after 16 weeks' gestation.[85] The alternative subcutaneous heparin does not give adequate protection in the low doses that have been used so far. Furthermore, even subcutaneous heparin therapy has the risk of bone demineralization. In the future, subcutaneous LMWH in high doses (e.g. enoxaparin 1 mg/kg twice daily), as has been discussed above for the acute treatment of thromboembolism, may prove to be the best treatment, and clinical trials of such therapy are in progress.

Use of the minimum dose of warfarin maintaining an international normalized ratio (INR) no greater than 3 probably decreases the teratogenic and abortion risks of warfarin[86,87] without any increase in the risk of thromboembolism.[88]

At 37 weeks, when the risk of bleeding in the warfarinized fetus in association with labour seems to be too great, the patient should be admitted to hospital and given continuous intravenous heparin. The aim should be to achieve a heparin level of 0.6–1.0 units per ml as assayed by protamine sulphate neutralization,[89] or to double the APTT when compared to control. It is believed that the clotting system of the fetus will return to normal after warfarin has been withheld for about 1 week. At that time, maternal heparin therapy should be reduced to give a heparin level of less than 0.2 units per ml and labour should be induced. If the patient inadvertently goes into labour taking warfarin, she should be given vitamin K to reverse the action of warfarin in the fetus and started on heparin therapy as above. In extreme cases, vitamin K has been given intramuscularly to the fetus in utero by transamniotic injection.[90] After delivery, because of the risk of maternal post-partum haemorrhage, the patient should continue to receive heparin for about 7 days; then warfarin may be recommenced.

An alternative approach to anticoagulation in the early part of pregnancy was that of Iturbe-Alessio et al.[86] in Mexico. They discontinued warfarin in 35 women as soon as they reported with pregnancy and substituted subcutaneous heparin 5000 units b.d. until the end of the 12th week. At this stage warfarin was recommenced to be replaced by heparin at the end of pregnancy. Ten thousand units of heparin per day is a very low dose in pregnancy. Our policy is to use an adjusted dose continuous heparin infusion in patients who wish to avoid warfarin at this crucial period in organogenesis and because of the abortion risk.

Conclusion

The use of anticoagulant drugs in pregnancy depends on the indication for the treatment. For established thromboembolism, heparin intravenous and then subcutaneous is the preferred treatment for the majority of patients. For thromboprophylaxis, high risk patients receive subcutaneous heparin throughout pregnancy; low risk patients receive antiplatelet drugs antenatally, and subcutaneous heparin in labour and for 6 weeks postnatally. For patients with artificial heart valves warfarin is the preferred treatment for the majority of pregnancy. High dose intravenous heparin should be substituted well before delivery and can also be given during organogenesis and because of the abortion risk.

Declaration of interest

Dr de Swiet has received research and travel funding from Rhone-Poulenc Rorer, the manufacturers of enoxaparin.

References

1 Drife J. *Why mothers die: Report on confidential enquiries into maternal deaths in the United Kingdom 1994–1996*. Department of Health, Welsh Office Scottish Office Department of Health Department of Health and Social Services Northern Ireland. London: The Stationery Office Ltd, 1998.
2 Sturridge F, de Swiet M, Letsky E. The use of low molecular weight heparin for thromboprophylaxis in pregnancy. *Br J Obstet Gynaecol* 1994; **101**: 69–71.
3 Gillis S, Shushan A, Eldor A. Use of low molecular weight heparin for prophylaxis and treatment of thromboembolism in pregnancy. *Int J Gynecol Obstet* 1992; **39**: 297–301.
4 Nelson-Piercy C, Letsky EA, de Swiet M. Low-molecular-weight heparin for obstetric thromboprophylaxis: Experience of sixty-nine pregnancies in sixty-one women at high risk. *Am J Obstet Gynecol* 1997; **176**: 1062–8.
5 Thompson AJ, Walker ID, Greer IA. Low-molecular-weight heparin for immediate management of thromboembolic disease in pregnancy. *Lancet* 1998; **352**: 1904.

6 Melissari E, Parker CJ, Wilson NV. Use of low molecular weight heparin in pregnancy. *Thromb Haemost* 1992; **68**: 652–6.
7 Hunt BJ, Doughty H-A, Majumdar G *et al.* Thromboprophylaxis in low molecular weight heparin (Fragmin) in high risk pregnancies. *Thrombos Haemost* 1997; **1**: 39–43.
8 Haas S. The role of low molecular weight heparins in the prevention of venous thromboembolism in surgery with special reference to Enoxaparin. *Haemostasis* 1996; **26**: 48–9.
9 Nelson-Piercy C. Low molecular weight heparin for obstetric thromboprophylaxis. *Br J Obstet Gynaecol* 1994; **101**: 6–8.
10 Gibson JL, Ekevall K, Walker I, Greer IA. Puerperal thrombophrophylaxis: comparison of the anti-Xa activity of enoxaparin and unfractionated heparin. *Br J Obstet Gynaecol* 1998; **105**: 795–7.
11 Low-molecular-weight heparins in orthopaedic surgery. *Drug Therapeut Bull*1993; 31: 37–8.
12 Hirsh J, Cade JF, O'Sullivan EF. Clinical experience with anticoagulant therapy during pregnancy. *BMJ* 1970; *I*: 270–3.
13 Hatjis CG. Heparin-induced thrombocytopenia in pregnancy. A case report. *J Reprod Med* 1984; **29**: 337–8.
14 Chong BH, Pitney WR, Castaldi PA. Heparin-induced thrombocytopenia: association of thrombotic complications with heparin-independent IgG antibody that induces thromboxane synthesis and platelet aggregation. *Lancet* 1982; **ii**: 1246–8.
15 Wolf H, Wick G. Antibodies interacting with, and corresponding binding site for heparin on human thrombocytes. *Lancet* 1986; **ii**: 222–3.
16 Cines DB, Kaywin P, Bina M, Tomaski A, Schrieber AD. Heparin-associated thrombocytopenia. *New Engl J Med* 1980; **303**: 788–95.
17 Calhoun BC, Hesser JW. Heparin-associated antibody with pregnancy: Discussion of two cases. *Am J Obstet Gynecol* 1987; **156**: 964–6.
18 Eichinger S, Kyrle PA, Brenner B. Thrombocytopenia associated with low-molecular-weight heparin. *Lancet* 1991; **337**: 1425–6.
19 LeCompte T, Luo SK, Stieltjes N, Lecrubier C, Samama MM. Thrombocytopenia associated with low-molecular-weight heparin. *Lancet* 1991; **338**: 1217.
20 Warkentin TE, Levine MN, Hirst J *et al.* Heparin-induced thrombocytopenia in patients treated with low-molecular-weight heparin or unfractionated heparin. *New Engl J Med* 1995; B: 1330–5.
21 Ajayi AA., Horn E H, Cooper J, Rubin PC. Effect of unfractionated heparin and the low molecular weight heparins, dalteparin and enoxaparin on platelet behaviour in pregnancy. *Br J Clin Pharma*; **35**: 90–1.
22 Tomsu M, Li TC, Preston F, Forrest ARW. Severe hyperlipidaemia in pregnancy related to the use of low-molecular-weight heparin – enoxaparin sodium (clexane). *J Obstet Gynaecol*1998; **18**: 83–4.
23 Blickstein D, Shaklai M, Inbal A. Warfarin antagonism by avocado. *Lancet* 1991; **337**: 914–15.
24 Bowler GM, Galloway DW, Meiklejohn BH, Macintyre CC. Sharp fall in blood pressure after injection of heparin containing chlorbutol. *Lancet* 1986; **i (8485)** 848–9.
25 Hull RD, Raskob GE, Rosenbloom D, Panju AA. Heparin for 5 days as compared with 10 days in the initial treatment of proximal venous thrombosis. *New Engl J Med* 1990; **322**: 1260–4.
26 Hull RD, Raskob GE, Pineo GF, Green D *et al.* Subcutaneous low-molecular-weight heparin compared with continuous intravenous heparin in the treatment of proximal-vein thrombosis. *New Engl J Med* 1992; **326**: 975–82.
27 Prandoni P, Lensing AWA, Buller HR *et al.* Comparison of subcutaneous low-molecular-weight with intravenous standard heparin in proximal deep-vein thrombosis. 1992; **339**: 441–3.
28 Pfeifer GW. The use of thrombolytic therapy in obstetrics and gynaecology. *Aust Ann Med* 1970; **19**(1): 28–31.
29 Bell WR, Meek AG. Guidelines for the use of thrombolytic agents. *New Engl J Med* 1979; **301**: 1266–70.
30 Pfeiffer GW. Distribution and placental transfer of 1411 streptokinase. *Aust Ann Med* (Suppl.) 1970; 17–18.
31 National Institute of Health. Thrombolytic therapy in treatment of pulmonary embolus. *BMJ* 1980; **280**: 1585–7.
32 Amias AG. Streptokinase cerebral vascular disease – and triplets. *BMJ* 1977; *I*: 1414–15.
33 Hall RJC, Young C, Sutton GC, Cambell S. Treatment of acute massive pulmonary embolism by streptokinase during labour and delivery. *Br Med J* 1972; **iv**: 647–9.

34 McTaggart DR, Ingram TG. Massive pulmonary embolism during pregnancy treated with streptokinase. *Med J Aust* 1977; **1**: 18–20.

35 Flute PT. Thrombolytic therapy. *Br J Hosp Med* 1976; **16**: 135–42.

36 Abbott A, Sibert JR, Weaver JB. Chondrodysplasia punctata and maternal warfarin treatment. BMJ 1977; **i**: 1639–40.

37 Becker MH, Genieser NB, Finegold M. Chondrodysplasia punctata: is maternal warfarin therapy a factor? *Am J Dis Child* 1975; **129**: 356–9.

38 Kerber IJ, Warr OS3, Richardson C. Pregnancy in a patient with a prosthetic mitral valve. Associated with a fetal anomaly attributed to warfarin sodium. *JAMA* 1968; **203**: 223–5.

39 Pettifor JM, Benson R. Congenital malformations associated with the administration of oral anticoagulants during pregnancy. *J Pediatr* 1975; **86**: 459–62.

40 Shaul WL, Emery H, Hall JG. Chondrodysplasia punctata and maternal warfarin use during pregnancy. *Am J Dis Child* 1975; **129**: 360–2.

41 Cox DR, Martin L, Hall BD. Asplenia syndrome after fetal exposuure to warfarin. *Lancet* 1977; **ii**: 1134.

42 O'Donnell D, Sevitz H, Seggie JL, Meyers AM, Botha JR, Myburgh JA. Pregnancy after renal transplantation. *Aust N Z J Med* 1985; **15**: 320–5.

43 Villasanta U. Thromboembolic disease in pregnancy. *Am J Obstet Gynecol* 1965; 93: 142–60.

44 Venous thromboembolism and anticoagulants in pregnancy. *BMJ* 1975; **ii**: 421–2.

45 Shaul WL, Hall JG. Multiple congenital anomalies associated with anticoagulants. *Am J Obstet Gynecol* 1977; **127**: 191–8.

46 Smith MF, Cameron MD. Warfarin as teratogen. *Lancet* 1979; *I*: 727.

47 Chen WWC, Chan CS, Lee PK, Wang RY, Wong VC. Pregnancy in patients with prosthetic heart valves: An experience with 45 pregnancies. *Q J Med* 1982; **51**: 358–65.

48 Chong MK, Harvey D, de Swiet M. Follow-up study of children whose mothers were treated with warfarin during pregnancy. *Br J Obstet Gynaecol* 1984; **91**: 1070–3.

49 de Swiet M, Letsky E, Mellows H. Drug treatment and prophylaxis of thromboembolism in pregnancy. In: Lewis P, ed. *Therapeutic problems In pregnancy.* Lancaster: MTPress, 1977, pp. 81–9.

50 Li TC, Smith ARB, Duncan SLB. Feto-maternal haemorrhage complicating warfarin therapy during pregnancy. *J Obstet Gynaecol* 1990; **10**: 4001–2.

51 Brambel C E, Hunter R E. Effect of dicoumarol on the nursing infant. *Am J Obstet Gynecol* 1950; **59**: 1153–9.

52 Orme ML, Lewis PJ, de Swiet M *et al.* May mothers given warfarin breast-feed their infants? *BMJ* 1977; **1**: 1564–5.

53 Eckstein HB, Jack B. Breast feeding and anticoagulant therapy. *Lancet* 1970; *I*: 672–3.

54 Oakley CM, Hawkins DF. Pregnancy in patients with prosthetic heart valves. *BMJ* 1983; **287**: 358.

55 Hirsh J. Heparin. *New Engl J Med* 1991; **324**: 1565–74.

56 Bonnar J. Thromboembolism in obstetric and gynaecological patients. In: Nicolaides AN, ed. *Thromboembolism aetiology, advances in prevention and management.* Lancaster: MTPress, 1975, pp. 311–34.

57 de Swiet M, Fidler J, Howell R, Letsky E. Thromboembolism in pregnancy. In: Jewell DP, ed. *Advanced medicine.* London: Pitman Medical, 1981, pp. 309–17.

58 Hill NCW, Hill JG, Sargent JM, Taylor CG, Bush PV. Effect of low dose heparin on blood loss at caesarean section. *BMJ* 1988; **296**: 1505–6.

59 Anderson DR, Ginsberg JS, Burrows R, Brill-Edwards P. Subcutaneous heparin therapy during pregnancy: a need for concern at the time of delivery. *Thromb Haemost* 1991; **65**: 1505–6.

60 Letsky E. Haemostasis and epidural anaesthesia. *Int J Obstet Anesth* 1991; **1**: 51–4.

61 Crawford JS. Crawford JS, eds. *Principles and practice of obstetric anaesthesia.* Oxford: Blackwell Scientific Publications, 1978, pp. 182–3.

62 Wysowski DK, Talarico L, Bacsanyi J, Botstein. P. Spinal and epidural hematoma and low-molecular-weight heparin. *New Engl J Med* 1998; **338**: 1774–4.

63 Badaracco MA, Vessey M. Recurrence of venous thromboembolism disease and use of oral contraceptives. *BMJ* 1974; *I*: 215–17.

64 Department of Health and Social Security. *Report on confidential enquiries into maternal deaths in England and Wales 1979–1981. 10.* London: HMSO, 1986.

65 Lowe GDO, Cooke T, Dewar EP. Thromboembolic risk factors (THRIFT) risks of and prophylaxis for venous thromboembolism in hospital patients. *BMJ* 1992; **305**: 567–74.

66 The Royal College of Obstetricians and Gynaecologists. *Report of the RCOG Working Party on Prophylaxis against thromboembolism in gynaecology and obstetrics.* London, Chameleon Press Ltd, 1995.

67 Avioli LV. Heparin-induced osteopenia: an appraisal. *Adv Exp Med Biol* 1975; **52**: 375–87.
68 Jaffe MD, Willis PW. Multiple factures associated with long-term sodium heparin therapy. *JAMA* 1965; **193**: 152–4.
69 Squires JW, Pinch LW. Heparin induced spinal fractures. *JAMA* 1979; **241**: 2417–18.
70 Griffith GC, Nichols G, Asher JD. Heparin osteoporosis. *JAMA* 1965; **193**: 91–4.
71 Griffiths HT, Liu DTY. Severe heparin osteoporosis in pregnancy. *Postgrad Med J* 1984; **60**: 424–5.
72 Dahlman TC. Osteoporotic fractures and the recurrence of thromboembolism during pregnancy and the puerperium in 184 women undergoing thromboprophylaxis with heparin. *Am J Obstet Gynecol* 1993; **168**: 1265–70.
73 Dahlman TC, Sjoberg HE, Hellgren M, Bucht E. Calcium homeostasis in pregnancy during long-term heparin treatment. *Br J Obstet Gynaecol* 1992; **99**: 412–16.
74 Misra R, Anderson DC. Providing the fetus with calcium. *BMJ* 1991; **300**: 1220–1.
75 Dahlman TC, Lindvall N, Hellgren M. Osteopenia in pregnancy during long-term heparin treatment: A radiological study postpartum. *Br J Obstet Gynaecol* 1990; **97**: 221–8.
76 Ginsberg JS, Kowalchuk. G. HJ, Brill-Edwards P, Burrows R, Coates G, Webber C. Heparin effect on bone density. *Thromb Haemost* 1990; **64**: 286–9.
77 Christiaens GCML, Nieuwenhuis HK. Heparin-Induced Skin Necrosis. *New Engl J Med* 1996; **335**: 715.
78 Ojukwu C, Jenkinson SD, Obeid D. Deep vein thrombosis in pregnancy and heparin hypersensitivity. *Br J Obstet Gynaecol* 1996; **103**: 934–6.
79 Canova CR, Fischler MP, Reinhart WH. Effect of low-molecular-weight heparin on serum potassium. *Lancet* 1997; **349**: 1447–8.
80 Lao TT, de Swiet M, Letsky E, Walters BNJ. Prophylaxis of thromboembolism in pregnancy: an alternative. *Br J Obstet Gynaecol* 1985; **92**: 202–6.
81 Thromboembolic Risk Factors (THRIFT) Consensus Group. Risk of and prophylaxis for venous thromboembolism in hospital patients. *BMJ* 1992; **305**: 567–74.
82 Antiplatelet Trialists' Collaboration. Collaborative overview of randomised trials of antiplatelet therapy – III: Reduction in venous thrombosis and pulmonary embolism by antiplatelet prophylaxis among surgical and medical patients. *BMJ* 1994; **308**: 235–46.
83 CLASP Collaborative Group. CLASP: a randomised trial of low-dose aspirin for the prevention and treatment of pre-eclampsia among 9364 pregnant women. *Lancet* 1994; **343**: 619–29.
84 Tan J, de Swiet M. Use of aspirin for obstetric thromboprophylaxis in low risk women. *J Obstet Gynaecol* 1998; **18**: S60.
85 Sahul WL, Hall JG. Multiple congenital anomalies associated with oral anticoagulants. *Am J Obstet Gynecol* 1977; **127**: 191–8.
86 Iturbe-Alessio I, Fonseca M, Mutchinik O, Santos MA, Zajartas A, Salazar E. Risks of anticoagulant therapy in pregnant women with artificial heart valves. *New Engl J Med* 1986; **315**: 1390–3.
87 Javares T, Coto EO, Maiques V, Rincon A, Such M, Caffarena JM. Pregnancy after heart valve replacement. *Int J Cardiol* 1984; **5**: 731–3.
88 Saour JN, Sieck JO, Mamo LA, Gallus AS. Trial of different intensities of anticoagulation in patients with prosthetic heart valves. *New Engl J Med* 1990; **322**: 428–32.
89 Dacie J. *Practical haematology*. Edinburgh: Churchill Livingstone, 1975, pp. 413–14.
90 Larsen JF, Jacobsen B, Holm HH, Pedersen JF, Mantoni M. Intrauterine injection of vitamin K before delivery during anticoagulant treatment of the mother. *Acta Obstet Gynecol Scand* 1978; **57**: 227–30.

5 Treatment of cardiovascular diseases

HELEN E HOPKINSON

Key points

- Angiotensin-coverting enzyme inhibitors and angiotensin II receptor antagonists are contraindicated in pregnancy.

- Beta-blockers are safe antihypertensive agents for use in the third trimester but can cause growth retardation if given throughout pregnancy.

- Methyldopa is a safe antihypertensive drug for use throughout pregnancy.

- The commonest arrhythmia in pregnancy is supraventricular tachycardia.

- Adenosine can be used to terminate supraventricular tachycardia in pregnancy and is safe in patients known to have an accessory conduction pathway.

- A beta-blocker may be preferable to verapamil for maternal SVT because there are fewer occurrences of fetal bradycardia.

- Digoxin is safe and effective for atrial fibrillation but toxic maternal levels can be fatal to the fetus.

Introduction

Pregnant women may require drug treatment for chronic cardiovascular disease which antedates the pregnancy, or for disease which develops or merits treatment for the first time in pregnancy. Broadly speaking the disorder will be either hypertension or a dysrhythmia. Heart failure is rare in pregnancy and requires specialist assessment and management beyond the scope of this chapter.

Several antihypertensive agents are safe and effective in pregnancy. A recent meta-analysis of antihypertensive drugs in pregnancy showed a reduction in perinatal death rate and in severe maternal hypertension, but no effect on intrauterine growth retardation or the development of pre-eclampsia in women with essential hypertension.[1] Therefore, the purpose of treatment remains to protect the mother from disasters such as intracerebral haemorrhage, and possibly to delay the need for delivery, but the prescriber's concern (and usually the mother's) is to avoid harmful fetal effects.

Hypertension

Angiotensin-converting enzyme inhibitors

Young patients with essential hypertension are often prescribed an angiotensin-converting enzyme (ACE) inhibitor once daily for ease of compliance and because there are few side effects. This is especially so in diabetic patients with microalbuminuria or nephropathy in whom ACE inhibitors provide an additional renoprotective effect. These drugs are contraindicated in pregnancy: oligohydramnios, fetal anuria and stillbirth have been reported.[2-7] ACE inhibitors limited to the first trimester do not seem to present a significant risk to the fetus.[8-11] Nevertheless, women taking these who are contemplating pregnancy should be changed to one of the alternatives below which have been more fully evaluated.

Angiotensin II receptor antagonists should not be prescribed in pregnancy because there is insufficient experience of their use in this situation.

Methyldopa

Methyldopa is regarded as a safe antihypertensive drug for use throughout pregnancy.[12] It crosses the placenta and is found in cord blood at similar concentration to that in the mother.[13] It reduces systolic blood pressure in neonates,[14] but there have been no reports of adverse fetal effects. Data for over 7 years of paediatric follow-up of infants, whose mothers were treated in pregnancy with methyldopa for hypertension or pre-eclampsia, show no evidence of any long-term abnormalities in infant development.[15]

66

Maternal side effects of methyldopa are manifestations of the drug's central nervous depressant action, and include drowsiness, depression, and postural hypotension. These may result in treatment being stopped in some individuals. Despite this, methyldopa remains a first-line drug for essential hypertension in the months before conception, and for antihypertensive treatment started during pregnancy.

Beta-blockers

Beta-adrenergic blocking agents are widely used in pregnancy for treating hypertension. They are effective, and many have been evaluated in clinical trials, although only two such trials had placebo controls.[16,17] Early anecdotal and retrospective reports of fetal complications and death associated with propranolol were not confirmed in prospective controlled studies. Beta-blockers cross the placenta and may cause a harmless lowering of fetal heart rate, but cardiotocographic reactivity is not affected by atenolol.[18] The effect of fetal beta-blockade may be important for very low birthweight babies, but a randomized study comparing maternal treatment with labetalol or hydralazine showed no difference in outcome for very low birthweight infants.[19] Fetal hydrops, bradycardia, and hypoglycaemia is occasionally still reported with chronic maternal beta-blockade.[20]

If treatment with atenolol is commenced before 28 weeks' gestation, gestationally adjusted birthweight is reduced,[21,22] but there is no evidence of persistent effects on infant growth.[23] Reported effects on fetal growth vary between different beta-blockers, and there is inconsistency between different trials using the same drug.[24-26] Maternal benefits in addition to the antihypertensive effect have been documented, although again the results of trials are conflicting. Treatment with atenolol,[16] acebutolol,[27] and labetalol,[28-30] has been associated with a decreased incidence of proteinuria later on, and even an improvement of pre-existing proteinuria. Beta-blockers are better tolerated than methyldopa, and a placebo-controlled, double-blind trial of atenolol[16] showed no difference between the treatment groups in maternal symptoms which could have been attributed to beta-blockers. In summary, beta-blockers are safe antihypertensive for use in the third trimester, and no single beta-blocker has been shown to be superior. However, if treatment is to be commenced before 28 weeks, methyldopa should be the first choice.

Calcium channel antagonists

Calcium channel antagonists – namely nifedipine, nicardipine, nitrendipine, and isradipine – have been shown to decrease blood pressure in pregnancy and to control antenatal and post-partum hypertension.[31-34] In acute severe hypertension nifedipine can be given orally or sublingually as an alternative to a parenteral drug; it has a relatively quick onset of action. However, there have been case reports of serious hypotensive reactions when nifedipine is given to women who are also receiving magnesium sulphate.[35] The only placebo-controlled trial of a calcium antagonist showed a significant hypotensive effect of isradipine in hypertensive pregnancy, but a sub-group analysis suggested that the drug was not effective if proteinuria was present.[34] There were no adverse fetal effects of isradipine in this study.[34] A prospective cohort study of patients contacting teratogen information services in Canada showed no increase in fetal malformation with exposure to calcium antagonists in the first trimester.[36]

Nimodipine is a selective cerebral vasodilator commonly used in the management of subarachnoid haemorrhage to prevent cerebral vasospasm. Its use in pre-eclampsia is also associated with maternal cerebral vasodilation[38] and reversal of cerebral vasospasm in eclampsia has also been reported.[39,40]

Diurectics

Diuretic agents are effective antihypertensives that are widely prescribed in the general population. They reduce effective circulating volume which is theoretically disadvantageous in women with hypertensive disease in pregnancy, as their intravascular volume may already be reduced.[41] Further depletion may seriously compromise uteroplacental blood flow, which in many cases will already be impaired. However, an overview of the use of mainly thiazide diuretics in pregnancy showed no adverse fetal effects.[42] In practice in the antenatal clinic, diuretics are not used for hypertensive diseases or simple oedema, but are reserved for the treatment of heart failure.

Prazosin

Prazosin is an alpha-adrenoceptor blocker which has been used in pregnancy as second-line antihypertensive treatment, usually in combination with a beta-blocking agent. Such a regimen led to improved blood pressure control in severe hypertension using prazosin with oxprenolol.[43] Fetal malformation has not been reported, although most experience is of its use later in pregnancy. The bioavailability of prasozin is increased during pregnancy,[44] so small doses (0.5 mg) should be used with appropriate precautions taken against first-dose hypotension.

Hydralazine

Hydralazine is another vasodilator that is an effective second-line antihypertensive when it is used in conjucntion with methyldopa or beta-blockers. Maternal compensatory tachycardia can be controlled with beta-blockade, but headache and facial flushing are less well tolerated. There are rare reports of neuropathy and lupus-like syndromes associated with hydralazine. Fetal problems are also rare, but neonatal thrombocytopenia has been recorded and linked to the use of hydralazine in the mother.

Drugs for hypertensive emergencies

The treatment for uncontrolled hypertension and pre-eclampsia is delivery. Nevertheless, blood pressure must be controlled in labour or before anaesthesia. An epidural anaesthetic is useful in this context but, according to the condition of the patient, either quick acting oral or parenteral drugs will be required.

- *Magnesium sulphate* is now the drug of choice for recurrent seizure prevention in eclampsia,[45] and is superior to phenytoin for primary seizure prevention in pre-eclampsia.[46] Caution is necessary in patients treated with a calcium antagonist, since neuromuscular blockade has been reported with a therapeutic magnesium concentration.[47] Magnesium sulphate may have some hypotensive effect itself[48] but the clinical use remains in seizure prevention.
- *Nifedipine* has already been described. It is absorbed readily via the sublingual route in acute severe hypertension.
- *Hydralazine* is effective given parenterally by bolus injection or infusion[49] but it takes upto 40 minutes to act. The maternal side effects may interfere with interpretation of the patient's condition.
- *Sodium nitroprusside* is administered parenterally and is recommended only for short-term use in the intensive care situation.
- *Ketanserin* is a selective serotonin2 receptor antagonist with mild alpha1–adrenoceptor antagonist activity. It was shown to be as

effective as hydralazine in lowering blood pressure in severe hypertension between 26 and 32 weeks' gestation. Ketanserin was effective more quickly and did not cause tachycardia.[50] There were no reports of adverse fetal effects with ketanserin.

Antiarrhythmic agents

The commonest arrhythmia in pregnancy, as in young people in general, is supraventricular tachycardia. It is important to exclude previously undetected disorders such as valvar heart disease and, even in apparently healthy pregnancy, the development of supraventricular tachycardia can occasionally be the first sign of pulmonary embolism. The ocurrence of an arrhythmia in pregnancy requires hospital assessment and management, preferably by doctors with experience in medical obstetrics. Prophylactic antiarrhythmic therapy is given for the same indications as in the nonpregnant state.

Adenosine

Adenosine given intravenously is used to restore sinus rhythm in paroxysmal supraventricular tachycardias when conventional nonpharmacological manoeuvres have failed. Adenosine is an endogenous nucleoside which transiently suppresses atrioventricular node conduction, and is safe to use in arrhythmias associated with accessory conduction pathways (e.g. Wolff–Parkinson–White syndrome). Its rapid onset of action and extremely short half-life support the expectation that the drug is safe in pregnancy, but experience is limited. There are several individual reports of successful and apparently safe use of adenosine for maternal supraventricular tachycardia in pregnancy[51–54] without effect on fetal cardiac rhythm.[55] A retrospective postal survey of North American obstetricians confirmed overall safety and efficacy for rapid termination of maternal supraventricular tachycardia in pregnancy.[56]

Adenosine administered direct to the fetus in utero has been reported in cases of fetal supraventricular tachycardia with hydrops fetalis, resistant to transplacental therapy.[57,58]

Digoxin

Digoxin is the drug of choice for the control of maternal atrial flutter or fibrillation. It is safe and effective, and there have been no

70

reports of teratogenicity. Digoxin crosses the placenta freely, and toxicity in the mother can be fatal to the fetus. Renal clearance increases as gestation advances, so the monitoring of levels is advisable and dose increments may be required. Digoxin has also been used successfully to control supraventricular tachycardia in the fetus.[59–61]

Verapamil

Verapamil belongs to the family of calcium antagonist drugs but has a predominantly negative chronotropic action. Its use in pregnancy is controversial because of potential fetal bradycardia; this deserves mention because it is probably the most commonly prescribed drug in young patients for prophylaxis of paroxysmal supraventricular tachycardia. There have been no reports of teratogenicity, but verapamil has been used in only a few patients. If a patient requires prophylaxis during pregnancy, a beta-blocker may be preferable.[62]

Amiodarone

Amiodarone is an effective antiarrhythmic drug for the prophylaxis and control of tachyarrhythmias of either ventricular or supraventricular origin. The drug is not a first-line antiarrhythmic even outside pregnancy because of its side effects. Amiodarone has a high iodine content which can lead to thyroid dysfunction in the mother and potentially in the fetus. Other common side effects include reversible corneal microdeposits, and photosensitivity.

Experience of the use of amiodarone in pregnancy is limited.[63,64] Both transient neonatal hyperthyroidism and hypothyroidism have been reported.[65] The drug is reserved for severe dysrhythmias resistant to other treatments. Fetal bradycardia may result from combination treatment especially with beta-blockers.[65] Amiodarone has also been used successfully to treat fetal tachyarrhythmia *in utero*, with resolution of hydrops and subsequent live birth.[66]

Prevention of pre-eclampsia

Aspirin

It has long been known that platelets are involved in the pathogenesis of pre-eclampsia and several small studies suggested that aspirin could prevent pre-eclampsia in those at risk of the condition.[67] However, two large and well-designed studies using 60 mg per day of aspirin have failed to confirm this early promise. In primigravid women, aspirin reduced the occurrence of pre-eclampsia from 6.3% to 4.6% compared with placebo, but placental abruption was increased seven-fold in the aspirin group, from 0.1% to 0.7%.[68] When women were studied in their second pregnancy, who had experienced pre-eclampsia in their first, aspirin did not influence the occurrence of pre-eclampsia: 6.7% in the aspirin group and 7.6% in the placebo group. On the basis of these findings, aspirin cannot be recommended for the routine prevention of pre-eclampsia.[69]

A small randomized, placebo-controlled trial of ketanserin and aspirin versus aspirin alone in the prevention of pre-eclampsia was performed in a mixed race African population of women with hypertension diagnosed before 20 weeks of pregnancy. This showed a benefit of ketanserin in reducing the incidence of pre-eclampsia (relative risk 0.15).[70]

References

1 Rey E, LeLorier J, Burgess E, Lange IR, Leduc L. Report of the Canadian Hypertension Society Consensus Conference: 3 Pharmacologic treatment of hypertensive disorders in pregnancy. *Can Med Ass J* 1997; 157: 1245–54.

2 Guignard JP, Burgener F, Calame A. Persistent anuria in a neonate: a side effect of captopril? *Int J Paediatr Nephrol* 1981; 2: 133.

3 Rothberg AD, Lorenz R. Can captopril cause fetal and neonatal renal failure? *Paediatr Pharmacol* 1984; 4: 189–92.

4 Knott PD, Thorpe SS, Lamont CAR. Congenital renal dysgenesis, possibly due to captopril. *Lancet* 1989; i: 451.

5 Kreft-Jais C, Plouin PF, Tchobroutsky C, Boutry J. Angiotensin-converting enzyme inhibitors during pregnancy: a survey of 22 patients given captopril and 9 given enalapril. *Br J Obstet Gynaecol* 1988; 95: 420–2.

6 Martin RA, Jones KL, Mendoza A, Barr MJ, Benirschke K. Effect of ACE inhibition on the fetal kidney: decreased renal blood flow. *Teratology* 1992; 46: 317–21.

7 Bhatt-Mehta V, Deluga KS. Fetal exposure to lisinopril: neonatal manifestations and management. *Pharmacotherapy* 1993; 13: 515–18.

8 Steffensen FH, Nielson GL, Sorensen HT, Olesen C, Olsen J. Pregnancy outcome with ACE-inhibitor use in early pregnancy. *Lancet* 1998; 351: 596.

9 Yip S, Leung T, Fung HYM. Exposure to angiotensin-converting enzyme inhibitors during first trimester: is it safe to fetus? *Acta Obstet Gynaecol Scand* 1998; 77: 570–1.

10 Lip GYH, Churchill D, Beevers M, Auckett A, Beevers DG. Angiotensin-converting-enzyme inhibitors in early pregnancy. *Lancet* 1997; 350: 1446–7.

11 Anonymous. From the Center for Disease Control and Prevention: Postmarketing surveillance for angiotensin-converting enzyme inhibitor use during the first trimester of pregnancy-United States, Canada, Israel, 1987–1995. *JAMA* 1997; 277: 1193–4.

12 Redman CWG, Beilin LJ, Bonnar J. Treatment of hypertension in pregnancy with methyldopa: blood pressure control and side effects. *Br J Obstet Gynaecol* 1977; 84: 419–26.

13 Jones HMR, Cummings AJ, Setchell KDR, Lawson AM. A study of the deposition of alpha-methyldopa in newborn infants following its administration to the mothers for the treatment of hypertension during pregnancy. *Br J Clin Pharmacol* 1979; 7: 433–40.

14 Whitelaw A. Maternal methyldopa treatment and neonatal blood pressure. *BMJ* 1981; 283: 471.

15 Ounsted M, Cockburn J, Moar VA, Redman CWG. Maternal hypertension with superim-

posed pre-eclampsia: effects on child development at 71/2 years. *Br J Obstet Gynaecol* 1983; **90**: 644–9.

16 Rubin PC, Butters L, Clark DM *et al.* Placebo-controlled trial of atenolol in treatment of pregnancy-associated hypertension. *Lancet* 1983; **2**: 431–4.

17 Pickles CJ, Broughton-Pipkin F, Symonds EM. A randomised placebo controlled trial of labetalol in the treatment of mild to moderate pregnancy induced hypertension. *Br J Obstet Gynaecol* 1992; **99**: 964–8.

18 Rubin PC, Butters L, Clark DM *et al.* Obstetric aspects of the use in pregnancy-associated hypertension of the beta-adrenoceptor antagonist atenolol. *Am J Obstet Gynecol* 1984; **150**: 389–92.

19 Hjertberg R, Faxelius G, Belfrage P. Comparison of outcome of labetalol or hydralazine therapy during hypertension in pregnancy in very low birthweight infants. *Acta Obstet Gynaecol Scand* 1993; **72**: 611–15.

20 Crooks BNA, Deshpande SA, Hall C, Ward Platt MP, Milligan DWA. Adverse neonatal effects of maternal labetalol treatment. *Arch Dis Child Fetal Neonatal Ed* 1998; **79**: F150–1.

21 Butters L, Kennedy S, Rubin PC. Atenolol in essential hypertension during pregnancy. *BMJ* 1991; **301**: 587–9.

22 Lip GYH, Beevers M, Churchill D, Shaffer LM, Beevers DG. Effect of atenolol on birthweight. *Am J Cardiol* 1997; **79**: 1436–8.

23 Reynolds B, Butters L, Evans J, Adams T, Rubin PC. First year of life after the use of atenolol in pregnancy associated hypertension. *Arch Dis Child* 1984; **59**: 1061–3.

24 Fidler JA, Smith V, Fayers P, de Swiet M. Randomised controlled comparative study of methyldopa and oxprenolol in treatment of hypertension in pregnancy. *BMJ* 1983; **286**: 1927–30.

25 Gallery EDM, Saunders DM, Hunyor SN, Gyory AZ. Randomised comparison of methyldopa and oxprenolol for treatment of hypertension in pregnancy. *BMJ* 1979; **1**: 1591–4.

26 Dubois D, Petitcolas J, Temperville B, Klepper A, Catherine PH. Treatment of hypertension in pregnancy with beta-adrenoreceptor antagonists. *Br J Clin Pharmacol* 1982; **13**: 375S–8S.

27 Williams ER, Morrissey JR. A comparison of acebutolol with methyldopa in the hypertensive pregnancy. *Pharmacotherapy* 1983; **3**: 487–91.

28 Symonds EM, Lamming GD, Jadoul F, Broughton-Pipkin F. Clinical and biochemical aspects of the use of labetalol in the treatment of hypertension in pregnancy: comparison with methyldopa. *Excerpta Medica* 1982; 62–76(Abstract).

29 Walker JJ, Crooks A, Erwin L, Calder AA. Labetalol in pregnancy induced hypertension: fetal and maternal effects. *Excerpta Medica* 1982; 148–60(Abstract).

30 Michael CA. Use of labetalol in the treatment of severe hypertension during pregnancy. *Br J Clin Pharmacol* 1979; **8**: 211S–15S.

31 Chidress CH, Katz VL. Nifedipine and its indications in obstetrics and gynaecology. *Obstet Gynaecol* 1994; **83**: 616–24.

32 Carbonne B, Jannet D, Touboul C, Khelifati Y, Milliez J. Nicardipine treatment of hypertension during pregnancy. *Obstet Gynaecol* 1993; **81**: 908–14.

33 Allen J, Maigaard S, Forman A *et al.* Acute effects of nitrendipine in pregnancy-induced hypertension. *Br J Obstet Gynaecol* 1987; **94**: 222–6.

34 Wide-Swensson DH, Ingemarsson I, Lunell N *et al.* Calcium channel blockade (isradipine) in treatment of hypertension in pregnancy: a randomised placebo-controlled study. *Am J Obstet Gynaecol* 1995; **173**: 872–8.

35 Waisman GD, Mayorga LM, Camera MI, Vignolo CA, Martinotti A. Magnesium plus nifedipine: potentiation of hypotensive effect in pre-eclampsia? *Am J Obstet Gynecol* 1988; **159**: 308–9.

36 Magee LA, Schick B, Donnenfield AE *et al.* The safety of calcium channel blockers in human pregnancy: a prospective multicenter cohort study. *Am J Obstet Gynecol* 1996; **174**: 823–8.

37 Papatsonis DN, van Geijn HP, Ader HJ, Lange FM, Bleker OP, Dekker GA. Nifedipine and ritodrine in the management of preterm labor: a randomized multicenter trial. *Obstet Gynaecol* 1997; **90**: 230–4.

38 Belfort MA, Saade GR, Moise KJ *et al.* Nimodipine in the management of pre-eclampsia: maternal and fetal effects. *Am J Obstet Gynaecol* 1994; **171**: 417–24.

39 Horn EH, Filshie M, Kerslake RW, Jaspan T, Worthington BS, Rubin PC. Widespread cerebral ischaemia treated with nimodipine in a patient with eclampsia. *BMJ* 1990; **301**: 794.

40 Belfort MA, Carpenter RJ, Kirshon B, Saade GR, Moise KJJ. The use of nimodipine in a patient with eclampsia: colour flow Doppler demonstration of retinal artery relaxation. *Am J Obstet Gynaecol* 1993; **169**: 204–6.

41 Sibai BM, Abdella TM, Spinnato JA, Shower DC. Plasma volume findings in patients with mild pregnancy-induced hypertension. *Am J Obstet Gynaecol* 1983; **147**: 16–20.

42 Collins R, Yusuf S, Peto R. Overview of randomised trials of diuretics in pregnancy. *BMJ* 1985; **290**: 17–23.

43 Lubbe WF, Hodge JV. Combined alpha and beta receptor antagonism with prasozin and oxprenolol in control of severe hypertension in pregnancy. 1981; **94**: 169–72.

44 Rubin PC, Butters L, Low RA, Reid JL. Clinical pharmacological studies with prasozin during pregnancy complicated by hypertension. *Br J Clin Pharmacol* 1983; **16**: 543–7.

45 Eclampsia Trial Collaborative Group. Which anticonvulsant for women with eclampsia? Evidence from the Collaborative Eclampsia trial. *Lancet* 1995; **345**: 1455–63.

46 Lucas MJ, Leveno KJ, Cunningham FG. A comparison of magnesium sulphate with phenytoin for the prevention of eclampsia. *New Engl J Med* 1995; **333**: 201–5.

47 Ben-Ami M, Giladi Y, Shalev E. The combination of magnesium sulphate and nifedipine: a cause of neuromuscular blockade. *Br J Obstet Gynaecol* 1994; **101**: 262–3.

48 Idama T, Lindow SW. Magnesium sulphate: a review of clinical pharmacology applied to obstetrics. *Br J Obstet Gynaecol* 1998; **105**: 260–8.

49 Paterson-Brown S, Robson SC, Redfern N, Walkinshaw SA, de Swiet M. Hydralazine boluses for the treatment of severe hypertension in pre-eclampsia. *Br J Obstet Gynaecol* 1994; **101**: 409–13.

50 Bolte AC, van Eyck J, Strack van Schijndel RJM, van Geijn HP, Dekker GA. The haemodynamic effects of ketanserin versus dihydralazine in severe early-onset hypertension in pregnancy. *Br J Obstet Gynaecol* 1998; **105**: 723–31.

51 Podolsky SM, Varon J. Adenosine use during pregnancy. *Ann Emerg Med* 1991; **20**: 1027–28.

52 Afridi I, Moise KJ, Rokey R. Termination of supraventricular tachycardia with intravenous adenosine in a pregnant woman with Wolff–Parkinson–White syndrome. *Obstet Gynaecol* 1992; **80**: 481–83.

53 Mason BA, Ricci-Goodman J, Koos BJ. Adenosine in the treatment of maternal paroxysmal supraventricular tachycardia. *Obstet Gynaecol* 1992; **80**: 478–80.

54 Matfin G, Baylis P, Adams P. Maternal supraventricular tachycardia treated with adenosine. *Postgrad Med J* 1993; **69**: 661–2.

55 Adair RF. Fetal monitoring with adenosine administration. *Ann Emerg Med* 1993; **22**: 1925.

56 Elkayam U, Goodwin TM. Adenosine therapy for supraventricular tachycardia during pregnancy. *Am J Cardiol* 1995; **75**: 521–3.

57 Kohl T, Tercanli S, Kececioglu D, Holzgreve W. Direct fetal administration of adenosine for the termination of incessant supraventricular tachycardia. *Obstet Gynaecol* 1995; **85**: 873–4.

58 Blanch G, Walkinshaw SA, Walsh K. Cardioversion of fetal tachyarrhythmia with adenosine. *Lancet* 1994; **344**: 1646.

59 Harrigan JT, Kangos JT, Sikka A, et al. Successful treatment of fetal congestive heart failure secondary to tachycardia. *New Engl J Med* 1981; **304**: 1527–9.

60 Hsieh Y, Lee C, Chang C, Tsai H, Yeh L, Tsai C. Successful prenatal digoxin therapy for Ebstein's anomaly with hydrops fetalis. A case report. *J Reprod Med* 1998; **43**: 710–12.

61 Tikanoja T, Kirkinen P, Nikolajev K, Eresmaa L, Haring P. Familial atrial fibrillation with fetal onset. *Heart* 1998; **79**: 195–7.

62 Chow T, Galvin J, McGovern B. Antiarrhythmic drug therapy in pregnancy and lactation. *Am J Cardiol* 1998; **82**: 58I–62I.

63 Foster CJ, Love HG. Amiodarone in pregnancy. Case report and review of the literature. *Int J Cardiol* 1988; **20**: 307–16.

64 Ovadia M, Brito M, Hoyer GL, Marcus FI. Human experience with amiodarone in the embryonic period. *Am J Cardiol* 1994; **73**: 316–17.

65 Magee LA, Downar E, Sermer M, Boulton BC, Allen LC, Koren G. Pregnancy outcome after gestational exposure to amiodarone in Canada. *Am J Obstet Gynaecol* 1995; **172**: 1307–11.

66 Rey E, Duperron L, Gauthier R, Lemay M, Grignon A, LeLorier J. Transplacental treatment of tachycardia-induced fetal heart failure with verapamil and amiodarone: a case report. *Am J Obstet Gynaecol* 1985; **153**: 311–12.

67 Rubin PC. Aspirin and pre-eclampsia. *Curr Obstet Gynaecol* 1994; **4**: 166–9.

68 Sibai BM, Caritis S, Thom E. Prevention of pre-eclampsia with low dose aspirin in healthy, nulliparous pregnant women. *New Engl J Med* 1993; **329**: 1213–19.

69 CLASP Collaborative group. CLASP: a randomised trial of low dose aspirin for the prevention and treatment of pre-eclampsia among 9364 pregnant women. *Lancet* 1994; **343**: 619–29.

70 Steyn DW, Odendaal HJ. Randomised controlled trial of ketanserin and aspirin in prevention of pre-eclampsia. *Lancet* 1997; **350**: 1267–71.

6 Treatment of endocrine diseases

BILL HAGUE

Key points

- Thyroid, adrenal, and vasopressin replacement therapy should be continued throughout pregnancy and while breastfeeding, with appropriate monitoring.

- Calcitriol therapy in hypoparathyroid women will need to be increased during pregnancy, but requires careful readjustment early in the puerperium.

- Women on long-term steroid therapy require parenteral hydrocortisone during labour.

- Propylthiouracil is the drug of choice for the treatment of thyrotoxicosis during pregnancy and lactation.

- The dose of propylthiouracil can usually be reduced as pregnancy proceeds in women with Graves' disease, but may require to be increased in the puerperium.

- Thyroid storm during pregnancy requires urgent vigorous therapy.

- Investigation of Cushing's syndrome should not be delayed because of pregnancy, as there is a high risk of adrenal malignancy in such women. Bromocriptine and cabergoline can usually be stopped in women with microprolactinomas who become pregnant.

- Bromocriptine can be used to shrink a prolactinoma that enlarges during pregnancy.

- Bromocriptine and cabergoline should not be used for suppression of lactation in women with hypertension or pre-eclampsia.

Introduction

This chapter reviews the use of drugs in pregnancy in all the main areas of endocrine disorder with the exception of diabetes mellitus, which is dealt with separately in Chapter 10.

Drugs are used for both diagnosis and management of endocrine diseases. Diagnosis involves assessment of basal function of an endocrine gland, followed by tests to suppress or stimulate that gland. Further diagnostic measures may well include localization procedures. Medical management usually takes the form of either hormone replacement therapy in the situation of endocrine failure, or of suppressive therapy in the case of hyperfunction.

Diagnostic measures

Thyrotoxicosis

After diabetes, thyrotoxicosis is the most common endocrine problem developing in pregnancy, many of the signs mimicking those of normal pregnancy. Diagnosis depends on the measurement of pituitary thyrotrophin (TSH) which is suppressed in active disease. The use of the sensitive radioimmunometric assay (IRMA) for TSH has now virtually done away with the need for the TRH (thyrotrophin releasing hormone) test in the assessment of thyroid function, as a measure of pituitary TSH response. Doubts have been expressed about the use of TRH in early pregnancy because of its effect of producing smooth muscle contraction.[1] It may also exacerbate hypertension.[2] Other diagnostic measures in thyrotoxicosis include the use of ^{131}I-uptake measurement, a test totally contraindicated in ongoing pregnancy, because of the risk of fetal uptake of the isotope and subsequent thyroidal damage, although complete destruction of the thyroid has not been documented with the diagnostic dose.[3]

Adrenal disorders

Other less common problems presenting in pregnancy are the adrenal disorders which cause hypertension.

Phaeochromocytoma This tumour may be suspected when urinary excretion of catecholamines or their metabolites is raised. Pentolinium, a quaternary ammonium ganglion blocking compound, has been used as a diagnostic agent. Failure to reduce plasma catecholamine concentrations after intravenous injection of pentolinium 5 mg provides additional evidence for establishing the diagnosis,[4] but no experience of this test in pregnancy has been described. Localization procedures for phaeochromocytoma generally include computed tomography and magnetic resonance. The use of [^{131}I]-*met*-iodobenzylguanidine (MIBG) should be avoided in pregnancy because of the radiation risk to the fetal thyroid.

Conn's syndrome   Mineralocorticoid excess is rare but may be suspected in patients with hypertension and hypokalaemia. The hypertension is rarely severe, and full investigation may be postponed until after pregnancy, when localization procedures, such as the use of radiolabelled selenium cholesterol, may be used without fear of fetal compromise.

Cushing's syndrome   Though rare, glucocorticoid excess presenting in pregnancy is much more serious, and needs urgent investigation because of the high risk (10%) of malignancy of the adrenal cortex.[5] Dexamethasone crosses the placenta with suppression of the fetal pituitary–adrenal axis,[6] but in the doses used for diagnosis, this suppression is short-lived. The use of metyrapone is discussed later.

Pituitary disorders

Investigation of anterior pituitary endocrine pathology usually includes assessing the response to insulin-induced hypoglycaemia. The transient nature of the hypoglycaemia is without serious risk to the fetus. The usual precautions of having an intravenous line open, with hydrocortisone and dextrose drawn up ready, as well as using a smaller dose of insulin for patients suspected of hypopituitarism, apply in pregnancy as much as for the non-pregnant patient. Investigation of posterior pituitary function may include assessment of the response to desmopressin, a vasopressin analogue. Published reports of its use in humans have shown that, unlike the naturally-occurring hormone, there is little evidence of a uterotonic effect.[7]

Management : hormone replacement therapy

Hypothyroidism

Hypothyroidism is usually diagnosed and treated before pregnancy, as the hypothyroid state is often associated with infertility.

There is also a high risk of poor pregnancy outcome, prior to thyroid hormone replacement, including frequent spontaneous abortions, a doubled stillbirth rate, an increased incidence of premature labour, and subnormal neonatal neurological development.[8] An increased risk of congenital abnormality in the offspring of these patients has been questioned.[9] Thyroid hormone replacement is achieved with the use of L-thyroxine 100–200 µg/day as a single dose, monitoring response by the fall of the serum TSH concentration. In pregnancy, the dose of thyroxine can usually be maintained.[10] The important point is to monitor and treat according to the biochemistry rather than by clinical judgment. Assessment of thyroid function tests once in each trimester is usually sufficient. In the puerperium, any increase in thyroxine dose will need reduction again. There is no contraindication to breastfeeding.

Hypoadrenalism

As with hypothyroidism, adrenal insufficiency is usually diagnosed and treated before pregnancy is possible. Replacement therapy (hydrocortisone 20–30 mg/day, fludrocortisone 0.05–0.20 mg/day) is essential, but needs no alteration in pregnancy unless intercurrent stress/illness occurs, when increased or parenteral doses should be employed. The oestrogen-mediated rise in cortisol binding globulin during pregnancy does not seem to affect steroid requirements. There may be an increased incidence of small-for-gestational-age infants in Addison's disease;[11] it is not clear whether this is due to the disease or the therapy. No other complication, either fetal or maternal, has been associated with steroid replacement therapy. Breastfeeding is not a problem.

Hypopituitarism

Anterior pituitary deficiency states require thyroxine and corticosteroid replacement therapy as above, with the exception that fludrocortisone is not required, mineralocorticoid secretion being pituitary independent. Untreated, hypopituitarism has a high mortality for both fetus and mother.[12] Hypogonadotrophic states may require exogenous gonadotrophin or, more physiologically, pulsatile gonadotrophin releasing hormone therapy, to achieve ovulation. Once pregnancy is achieved, however, maintenance therapy is not necessary because of the gonadotrophin and sex steroid production by the fetoplacental unit. Lactation may be impaired because of prolactin deficiency.

Posterior pituitary failure is associated with diabetes insipidus, requiring the use of the vasopressin analogue desmopressin (dDAVP) (5–10 µg b.d.) as replacement. A review of 67 cases[13] showed that 58% of patients deteriorated during pregnancy. The mechanism for this is unclear but may reflect the increase in metabolic clearance of vasopressin in pregnancy. No ill effects of dDAVP in pregnancy have been reported apart from a small risk of increased uterine contractility from its oxytocin-like structure and activity.[14] This effect, however, is seen when dDAVP is used intravenously as a diagnostic agent rather than with the normal replacement regimen using nasal insufflation. dDAVP has 75 times less the oxytocic action of arginine vasopressin.

Hypoparathyroidism

Usually associated with the post-thyroidectomy state, but occasionally seen as part of an autoimmune diathesis or as a hormone resistant syndrome, hypoparathyroidism in the mother poses severe risks of neonatal rickets that may be fatal. Treatment with calcium (1600–2000 µg/day) and either vitamin D (1.25–2.5 mg/day) or dihydrotachysterol (250–1000 µg/day) is essential, with frequent monitoring of maternal Ca^{2+} and PO_4^{2-} to maintain normocalcaemia.[15] The vitamin D requirement increases two- to three-fold during pregnancy.[16] The use of calcitriol has been associated with fetal hypermineralization in one of twin fetuses.[17] In the puerperium, the requirement for calcium and vitamin D should be reassessed without delay; they may not be required at all.[18] In the normal woman, an insignificant amount of vitamin D is secreted in the breast milk,[19] but the high doses of vitamin D required in the lactating hypoparathyroid woman may cause neonatal hypervitaminosis.

Management: endocrine gland hyperfunction

Thyrotoxicosis

The mainstay of medical therapy of thyrotoxicosis are: propylthiouracil (PTU), carbimazole (CBZ), and its metabolite methimazole (MZ). PTU is less lipid soluble and more highly protein bound than CBZ or MZ, and is less well transferred into the breast milk[20] or, theoretically, across the placenta. No teratogenic effects have been reported for PTU or CBZ, but there have been five neonates recorded with a scalp defect, aplasia cutis, following maternal MZ therapy.[21] One study has suggested that maternal thyrotoxicosis may itself be associated with fetal malformation, and that the risk may be reduced by antithyroid drug therapy.[22] Perinatal mortality is also high in the untreated group with a high incidence of premature delivery, that can be reduced to normal with therapy.[23] Fetal hypothyroidism is a definite risk with all thionamide therapy, such that the lowest possible dose to maintain biochemical euthyroidism in the mother must be used, with (at least) bimonthly checks on the free thyroid hormone and TSH concentrations. Fetal goitre formation, however, is not dose related; it is affected by maternal antibody status and iodine intake. Intellectual development of children exposed *in utero* to antithyroid drugs is unaffected.[23]

Autoimmune thyrotoxicosis frequently improves during pregnancy so that the dose of drug may be reduced, while post partum a flare of overactivity is common,[24] requiring an increase in therapy. Women with autonomous toxic thyroid nodules are more difficult to treat during pregnancy, as use of antithyroid drugs will suppress the fetal thyroid without the associated presence of thyroid stimulating antibodies to counteract the effect. Beta-blocking drugs, such as propranolol, may be used to hold the situation until pregnancy is complete. (For a full discussion of beta-blockade, see Chapter 5.) Otherwise, hemithyroidectomy may be considered in the second trimester.

Other agents used to control thyrotoxicosis include potassium iodide and radioactive iodine. Potassium iodide, often used in preparation for thyroid surgery, is well recognized as a fetal goitrogen;[25] fetal goitre has been reported when the mother has received as little as 12 mg iodide per day. Radio-iodine (^{131}I) in therapeutic doses is liable to ablate the fetal thyroid, and also has the potential to induce maternal thyroid storm (see below). Paradoxically, the risk to the fetus is least in the first trimester before the fetal iodine trap is operational.[26]

In the light of the above, propylthiouracil is probably the drug of choice in both pregnancy and puerperium, with 100–150 mg/8 hours initially, and reducing to 50 mg/6–8 hours once the hyperthyroid state is controlled clinically and, more importantly, biochemically. The lowest possible maintenance dose should be used to maintain the free thyroxine in the high normal range. If thyrotoxicosis recurs or is not controlled, doses up to 600 mg/day in divided doses may be used. Failure of control may indicate the need for partial thyroidectomy, when propranolol (40 mg/6 hours) may be given to control residual symptoms prior to surgery.

Fetal and neonatal thyrotoxicosis may occur secondary to the transplacental passage of thyroid stimulating antibodies in the absence of maternal signs following thyroid ablation or, rarely, in maternal autoimmune hypothyroidism. Thionamide therapy has been used successfully to control the fetal thyrotoxicosis, with the fetal heart rate monitored as a guide to dose.[27] Intra-amniotic administration of thyroxine has been used in suspected fetal hypothyroidism,[28] but experience with this is limited, and careful screening and follow-up of such infants is needed.

Unrecognized thyrotoxicosis may lead rarely to the onset of thyroid storm, with the stress of an infection or, in the pregnant woman, of labour or operative delivery. This is a medical emergency with a high risk of morbidity and mortality to mother and fetus. Intravenous fluids, high doses of propylthiouracil (600–800 mg stat, 150–200 mg 4–6 hourly) followed one to two hours later by iodide therapy (KI 2–5 drops p.o., or NaI 0.5–1.0 g i.v., every 8 hours), dexamethasone (2 mg 6 hourly $\times$ 4), propranolol (20–80 mg p.o. or 1–10 mg i.v., every 4 hours), phenobarbitone (30–60 mg 6–8 hourly), oxygen and supportive therapy should be given, preferably in an intensive care or high dependency setting.[29] Treatment should be started without waiting for laboratory confirmation of hyperthyroidism.

Cushing's syndrome

Drugs used in the management of Cushing's syndrome include metyrapone, trilostane and aminoglutethimide, all of which block various points in the biosynthetic pathway of cortisol, and cyproheptadine, a serotonin antagonist which is used to suppress corticotrophin releasing hormone. Experience in the use of all these drugs in pregnancy is limited because of the rarity of the syndrome. Metyrapone has not been shown to have any adverse effects on fetus or mother in normal pregnancy.[30] Studies in baboons have shown an inhibition of surfactant release, although the offspring did not develop respiratory distress.[31] Metyrapone has been used successfully in Cushing's syndrome in pregnancy with survival of both mother and infant.[32] In a second report, however, the use of metyrapone coincided with the onset of severe preeclampsia at 26+ weeks gestation, and the fetus succumbed with a complication of premature delivery.[33] The link between the use of metyrapone, with its action of increasing 11–deoxycorticosterone (DOC) production, and the exacerbation of maternal hypertension in this case is not clear.

Trilostane, with its 3β-hydroxysteroid dehydrogenase antagonism, has been shown to inhibit placental progesterone production with the risk of abortion or premature labour,[36] and is therefore contraindicated in pregnancy. The use of aminoglutethimide and cyproheptadine has been reported in one case each,[35,36] but with limited data as to outcome. Ketoconazole is teratogenic and embryotoxic in animals, and should not be used in human pregnancy.

In view of the high proportion (10%) of adrenal malignancy among pregnant patients with Cushing's syndrome, active surgical and/or obstetric management has been recommended in the first and last trimesters, with metyrapone reserved for the difficult problems of the second trimester.[37] There are no data on the use of metyrapone in lactating women, although being lipid soluble, it is likely to be excreted into the breast milk.

Congenital adrenal hyperplasia

Few pregnancies have been described in women with congenital adrenal hyperplasia diagnosed in infancy.[38] Such patients may have had clitoral surgery and vaginal scarring. Those with 11β-hydroxylase deficiency may also be severely hypertensive. Adrenal suppression in these patients is achieved with replacement glucocorticoid and, in the case of salt-wasting 21–hydroxylase deficiency, with mineralocorticoid therapy, both of which should be maintained in pregnancy as for patients with hypoadrenalism. Women with late-onset congenital adrenal hyperplasia almost always have polycystic ovary syndrome, and often require adrenal suppression with glucocorticoids to allow ovulation to occur. Once pregnancy has been achieved in such patients, however, the glucocorticoid can be weaned without detriment to the mother or fetus.

Recently, treatment of the fetus with adrenal hyperplasia has been achieved by giving dexamethasone to the mother in the first and second trimesters to suppress fetal ACTH production; fetal adrenal androgen output is thus reduced with the associated masculinization of female genitalia.[39] Maternal risks associated with this therapy include hypertension, diabetes, and osteoporosis.

All women who have been taking prolonged steroid therapy for whatever reason should receive supplementary parenteral hydrocortisone 100 mg 6-hourly during labour or at the time of caesarean section to avoid the small risk of hypoadrenal crisis.

Phaeochromocytoma

The management of phaeochromocytoma in pregnancy is surgical, once control of the circulating catecholamine effects has been achieved with the use of alpha- and beta-adrenoceptor blocking agents.[40] Use of magnesium sulphate has also been advocated to aid control of vascular reactivity.[41]

Hyperprolactinaemia and acromegaly

Dopaminergic agents, such as bromocriptine or cabergoline, are the treatment of choice in the management of pathological hyperprolactinaemia, allowing ovulation and, in the case of pituitary micro- or macroadenomas, reduction of tumour size. They also have a place in the management of acromegaly in reducing growth hormone secretion, although this is not always so successful.

Bromocriptine has been used to suppress lactation. However, rare but serious complications, including myocardial infarction, hypertension, and stroke, have been reported following the use of bromocriptine for this purpose.[42] Bromocriptine and cabergoline should therefore not be used in women with hypertension or pre-eclampsia.

No ill effects to the fetus have been reported, either of women in whom ovulation was induced with bromocriptine, or of women given bromocriptine throughout pregnancy,[43] although there is evidence that bromocriptine, or an active metabolite, does cross the placenta.[44] Clinical experience of cabergoline in human pregnancy is still limited and the manufacturers recommend patients come off therapy prior to conception

The use of bromocriptine in pregnancy should be reserved for the small number of women who present with symptoms and signs of tumour expansion, in whom high resolution CT or MRI scanning confirms the diagnosis, and in whom immediate delivery is not practicable or desirable.[45] Treatment starts at 5 mg/day in divided doses, doubling daily over 3 days until symptoms resolve, or until the patient is taking 20 mg/day, or has developed side effects. Surgery is rarely necessary. Lactation in such patients is both suppressed and contraindicated, and early contraception must be considered.

As with Cushing's syndrome, acromegaly is rarely seen in pregnancy.[46] Dopaminergic therapy has been used and, theoretically, use of the somatostatin analogue octreotide could be considered if there was evidence of active progressive acromegaly, and surgery was thought to be contraindicated. The long-term use of octreotide in pregnancy has only been reported once in a woman with a TSH-adenoma with no apparent adverse effects on the neonate.[47]

Hyperparathyroidism

The treatment of symptomatic hyperparathyroidism in pregnancy is surgical. Fluid replacement may be necessary prior to operation, if the hypercalcaemia is severe.[48] Mild hypercalcaemia without symptoms may respond to phosphate and/or magnesium therapy. The neonate needs careful observation for signs of hypocalcaemia (secondary to parathormone suppression) which may present late in the postnatal period.

References

1 Reynolds JEF, ed. *Martindale: the extra pharmacopoeia*. London: Pharmaceutical Press, 1982, pp. 1276–7.

2 Borowski GD, Garofano CD, Rose LI, Levy RA. Blood pressure response to thyrotropin releasing hormone in euthyroid subjects. *J Clin Endocrinol Metab* 1984; **38**: 197–200.

3 Hays PM, Cruikshank DP. Hormonal therapy during pregnancy. In: Eskes TKAB, Finster M, eds. *Drug therapy during pregnancy*. London: Butterworths, 1985, pp. 110–60.

4 Brown MJ, Allison DJ, Jenner DA, Lewis PJ, Dollery CT. Increased sensitivity and accuracy of phaeochromocytoma diagnosis achieved by use of plasma-adrenaline estimations and a pentolinium-suppression test. *Lancet* 1981; **i**: 174–7.

5 Buescher MA, McClamrock HD, Adashi EY. Cushing syndrome in pregnancy. *Obstet Gynecol* 1992; **79**: 130–7.

6. Funkhouser JD, Peevy KJ, Mockridge PB, Hughes ER. Distribution of dexamethasone between mother and fetus after maternal administration. *Pediatr Res* 1978; **12**: 1053–6.

7 Ray JG. dDAVP use during pregnancy: an analysis of its safety for mother and child. *Obstet Gynecol Surv* 1998; **53**: 450–5.

8 Thomas R, Reid RL. Thyroid disease and reproductive dysfunction. *Obstet Gynecol* 1987; **70**: 789–98.

9 Montoro M, Collea JV, Frasier SN, Mestman JH. Successful outcome of pregnancy in women with hypothyroidism. *Ann Int Med* 1981; **94**: 31–4.

10 Girling JC, de Swiet M. Thyroxine dosage during pregnancy in women with primary hypothyroidism. *Br J Obstet Gynaecol* 1992; **99**: 368–70.

11 Osler M. Addison's disease and pregnancy. *Acta Endocrinol* 1962; **41**: 67–78.

12 Grimes HG, Brooks MH. Pregnancy in Sheehan's syndrome. Report of a case and review. *Obstet Gynecol Surv* 1980; **35**: 481–8.

13 Hime MC, Richardson JA. Diabetes insipidus and pregnancy. Case report, incidence, and review of the literature. *Obstet Gynecol Surv* 1978; **33**: 375–9.

14 Baylis PH, Thompson C, Burd J, Tunbridge WM, Snodgrass CA. Recurrent pregnancy induced polyuria and thirst due to hypothalamic diabetes insipidus: an investigation into possible mechanisms responsible for polyuria. *Clin Endocrinol* 1986; **24**: 459–66.

15 Montoro M, Mestman JH. How to manage parathyroid disease in the pregnant patient and neonate. *Contemporary Obstetrics and Gynaecology* 1981; **17**: 143–57.

16 Sadeghi-Nejad A, Wolfsdorf JI, Senior B. Hypoparathyroidism and pregnancy treatment with calcitriol. *JAMA* 1980; **243**: 254–5.

17 Salle BL, Berthezene F, Glorieux FH *et al.* Hypoparathyroidism during pregnancy: treatment with calcitriol. *J Clin Endocrinol Metab* 1981; **52**: 810–13.

18. Wright AD, Joplin GF, Dixon HG. Post-partum hypercalcaemia in treated hypoparathyroidism. *BMJ* 1969; **i**: 23–5

19 Beeley L. Drugs and breastfeeding. *Clin Obstet Gynaecol* 1986; **13**: 247–51.

20 Kampmann JP, Hansen JM, Johansen K, Helweg J. Propylthiouracil in human milk. *Lancet* 1980; **i**: 736–7.

21 Mujtaba O, Burrow GN. Treatment of hyperthyroidism in pregnancy with propylthiouracil and methimazole. *Obstet Gynecol* 1975; **46**: 282–6.

22 Momotani M, Ito K, Hamada N, Ban Y, Nishikawa Y, Mimura T. Maternal hyperthyroidism and congenital malformation in the offspring. *Clin Endocrinol* 1984; **20**: 695–700.

23 Burrow GN, Bartsocas D, Klatskin DH, Grunt JA. Children exposed in utero to propylthiouracil. Subsequent intellectual and physical development. *Am J Dis Child* 1968; **116**: 161–5.

24 Amino N, Miyai K, Yamamoto T *et al*. Transient recurrence of hyperthyroidism after delivery in Graves' disease. *J Clin Endocrinol Metab* 1977; **44**: 130–6.

25 Senior B, Chernoff HL. Iodide goiter in the newborn. *Pediatrics* 1971; **47**: 510–15.

26 Stouffer SS, Hamburger JT. Inadvertent ^{131}I therapy for hyperthyroidism in the first trimester of pregnancy. *J Nucl Med* 1976; **17**: 146–9.

27 Cove DH, Johnston P. Fetal hyperthyroidism: experience of treatment in four siblings. *Lancet* 1985; **i**: 430–2.

28 Lightner ES, Fismer DA, Giles H, Woolfenden J. Intra-amniotic injection of thyroxine (T4) to a human fetus. Evidence for conversion of T4 to reverse T3. *Am J Obstet Gynecol* 1977; **127**: 487–90.

29 Molitch M. Endocrine emergencies in pregnancy. *Baillière's Clin Endocrinol Metab* 1992; **6**: 167–91.

30 Heinen G, Buchheit M, Oertal W. Untersuchungen mit dem adrenostatikum SU4885 (Metopiron) in der schwangerschaft. *Klin Wochensch* 1963; **41**: 103–5.

31 Kling OR, Kotas RV. Endocrine influences on pulmonary maturation and the lecithin/sphingomyelin ratio in the fetal baboon. *Am J Obstet Gynecol* 1975; **121**: 664–8.

32 Gormley MJJ, Hadden DR, Kennedy TL, Montgomery DAD, Murnaghan GA, Sheridan B. Cushing's syndrome in pregnancy – treatment with metyrapone. *Clin Endocrinol* 1982; **16**: 283–93.

33 Connell JMC, Cordiner J, Davies DL, Fraser R, Frier BM, McPherson SG. Pregnancy complicated by Cushing's syndrome: potential hazard of metyrapone therapy. Case report. *Br J Obstet Gynaecol* 1985; **92**: 1192–5.

34 van der Spuy ZM, Jones DL, Wright CSW *et al*. Inhibition of 3β-hydroxysteroid dehydrogenase activity in first trimester human pregnancy with trilostane and WIN 32729. *Clin Endocrinol* 1983; **19**: 521–32.

35 Hanson TJ, Ballonoff LB, Northcutt RC. Aminoglutethimide and pregnancy. *JAMA* 1974; **230**: 963–4.

36 Aron DC, Schall AM, Sheeler LR. Cushing's syndrome and pregnancy. *Am J Obstet Gynecol* 1990; **162**: 244–52.

37 van der Spuy ZM, Jacobs HS. Management of endocrine disorders in pregnancy – Part II. *Postgrad Med J* 1984; **60**: 312–20.

38 Premawardhana LD, Hughes IA, Read GF, Scanlon MF. Longer term outcome in females with congenital adrenal hyperplasia (CAH): the Cardiff experience. *Clin Endocrinol Oxf* 1997; **46**: 327–32.

39 Mercado AB, Wilson RC, Cheng KC, Wei JQ, New MI. Prenatal treatment and diagnosis of congenital adrenal hyperplasia owing to steroid 21–hydroxylase deficiency. *J Clin Endocrinol Metab* 1995; **80**: 2014–20.

40 Lau P, Permezel M, Dawson P, Chester S, Collier N, Forbes I. Phaeochromocytoma in pregnancy. *Aust NZ J Obstet Gynaecol* 1996; **36**: 472–6.

41 James MF. Use of magnesium sulphate in the anaesthetic management of phaeochromocytoma: a review of 17 anaesthetics. *Br J Anaesth* 1989; **62**: 616–23.

42 Kulig K, Moore LL, Kirk M, Smith D, Stallworth J, Rumack B. Bromocriptine-associated headache: possible life-threatening sympathomimetic interaction. *Obstet Gynecol* 1991; **78**: 941–3.

43 Krupp P, Turkalj I. Surveillance of Parlodel (bromocriptine) in pregnancy and offspring. In: Jacobs HS, ed. *Prolactinomas and pregnancy*. Lancaster: MTP Press, 1984, pp. 45–50.

44 Bigazzi M, Ronga R, Lancranjan I *et al*. A pregnancy in an acromegalic woman during bromocriptine treatment: effects on growth hormone and prolactin in the maternal, fetal and amniotic compartments. *J Clin Endocrinol Metab* 1979; **48**: 9–12.

45 Bergh T, Nillius SJ. Prolactinomas in pregnancy. In: Jacobs HS, ed. *Prolactinomas and pregnancy*. Lancaster: MTP Press, 1984, pp. 51–5.

46 Herman-Bonert V, Seliverstov M, Melmed S. Pregnancy in acromegaly: successful therapeutic outcome. *J Clin Endocrinol Metab* 1998; **83**: 727–31.
47 Caron P, Gerbeau C, Pradayrol L, Simonetta C, Bayard F. Successful pregnancy in an infertile woman with a thyrotropin-secreting macroadenoma treated with somatostatin analog (octreotide). *J Clin Endocrinol Metab* 1996; **81**: 1164–8.
48 Clark D, Seeds JW, Cefalo RC. Hyperparathyroid crisis and pregnancy. *Am J Obstet Gynecol* 1981; **140**: 840–2.

7 Treatment of rheumatic diseases

MARGARET A BYRON

Key points

- In rheumatic diseases drugs might be required to enable a woman to become pregnant.

- Analgesics and anti-inflammatory agents are often self-prescribed.

- Paracetamol is safe in pregnancy and lactation.

- Indomethacin has major adverse effects in both preterm and term babies.

- NSAIDs used in pregnancy and lactation should be those with a short half-life and inactive metabolites – ibuprofen, for example.

- Prednisolone is safe in pregnancy and lactation.

- Sulphasalazine is safe in pregnancy and lactation.

- Gold and penicillamine are relatively safe in pregnancy but their doses should be reduced.

- Cytotoxic drugs should be discontinued 2–3 months before pregnancy.

- Azathioprine, cyclosporin, and steroids are relatively safe in pregnancy and might be needed to control the underlying disease.

Introduction

Musculoskeletal disorders are very common, accounting for nearly one-fifth of all consultations in primary care.[1] Some conditions, such as low back pain and carpal tunnel syndrome, may require treatment during pregnancy, and other specific rheumatological conditions, such as systemic lupus erythematosus, and rheumatoid arthritis, have their peak incidence in women of childbearing age.

An adequate explanation of the risks of any proposed treatment, with appropriate advice on contraception, is essential when treating women of childbearing age. In women with established rheumatic diseases, pregnancy may not occur or may not be carried to term without the use of drugs that suppress the disease. Adequate control of the disease also enables a woman to feel capable of bearing and raising children. There is a good chance of remission of rheumatoid arthritis during pregnancy, although for systemic lupus erythematosus aggressive treatment may continue to be necessary.[2] The use of drugs that pose the least threat to the fetus will minimize anxiety, should pregnancy occur.

Table 7.1 lists the drugs prescribed for rheumatic conditions; several reviews examine the effects of these drugs in pregnancy and lactation.[3,4,5] Analgesics and NSAIDs are most commonly pre-

Table 7.1   Drugs used for rheumatological conditions

Drug	Rheumatological condition
Analgesics	Soft tissue lesions
NSAIDs	Inflammatory arthritis
	Osteoarthritis
	Non-specific back pain
Disease-modifying antirheumatic drugs	
sulphasalazine	Rheumatoid arthritis
	Ankylosing spondylitis
antimalarials	Systemic lupus erythematosus
	Rheumatoid arthritis
gold salts	Rheumatoid arthritis
penicillamine	Psoriatic arthritis
Immunosuppresive drugs:	
cytotoxic agents	
methotrexate	Severe unremitting rheumatoid arthritis
cyclophosphamide	Systemic lupus erythematosus
azathioprine	Other connective tissue diseases
corticosteroids	Systemic lupus erythematosus
	Other connective tissue diseases
	Rheumatoid arthritis
cyclosporin	Severe unremitting rheumatoid arthritis
	Psoriatic arthritis
Biological agents	Rheumatoid arthritis – still
	experimental (see text)
anti-TNF etc.	

scribed, and also account for a large proportion of self-prescription (over-the-counter) drugs. A study in Cape Town showed that 29% of pregnant women self-prescribed and 60% did not know that certain medicines are unsafe in pregnancy.[6] It cannot therefore be assumed that women are always aware of the risks.

Analgesics

Analgesics are commonly prescribed and bought over the counter during pregnancy, especially paracetamol. This crosses the placenta easily but is not associated with fetal malformations.[3,4,7] Codeine is also safe in pregnancy, although a neonatal drug withdrawal syndrome has been described with codeine and dextropropoxyphene.[4] Even with established inflammatory arthritis, well motivated women with moderate symptoms may be managed with simple analgesics, paracetamol being the drug of choice.

Breastfeeding

Paracetamol is excreted in small amounts in breast milk but is a safe analgesic to use during lactation.[8] Although codeine is lipid soluble and might concentrate in breast milk, it is considered safe in breastfeeding.

Non-steroidal anti-inflammatory drugs (NSAIDs)

These are first-line agents in treating inflammatory polyarthritis. For soft tissue and degenerative conditions, anti-inflammatory drugs should be prescribed only for the short term. Analgesics should be used if possible. Anti-inflammatory drugs have been implicated in causing infertility by increasing the frequency of luteinized unruptured follicles.[9] How often this accounts for failure of ovulation is unclear.

Teratogenicity

Animal studies have linked a variety of skeletal and craniovertebral abnormalities with ingestion of large doses of salicylates during pregnancy. In humans several retrospective surveys have shown that significantly more mothers of malformed infants took salicylates regularly during pregnancy than mothers of normal infants.

These findings have not been corroborated in prospective studies.[10–13] The largest study, the Perinatal Collaborative Project in the United States, found that malformation rates were similar in the children of 35 418 women not exposed to aspirin, 9736 with intermediate exposure, and 5128 heavily exposed during the first four months of pregnancy.[14] Overall, therefore, the evidence suggests that salicylates used in recommended doses are unlikely to produce fetal malformation. Diflunisal, a salicylic acid derivative, has been shown to be teratogenic in animals at very high doses, but no such abnormalities have been reported in humans.[14]

Other NSAIDs have not been as well studied as aspirin. The only reports of fetal malformation in humans are two anecdotal case reports implicating indomethacin.[3]

There is little information on the newer anti-inflammatories, such as etodolac, nabumetone, or meloxicam, but no evidence of teratogenicity has been found with commonly prescribed propionic acid derivatives such as ibuprofen, ketoprofen, flurbiprofen, fenoprofen, and naproxen. Phenylbutazone is best avoided in pregnancy as it has been associated with chromosomal abnormalities in adults.[3,4]

Fetal growth retardation

A survey from Sydney showed that long-term ingestion of aspirin was associated with an increased incidence of stillbirth and reduced birthweight compared with that of controls.[12] Most of the aspirin preparations ingested, however, were compounds containing substances such as phenacetin and caffeine, and were taken in large doses. Data from the United States showed no significant effect of aspirin ingestion on birthweight and perinatal mortality.[10,12,13] There is no convincing evidence that indomethacin or other non-steroidal anti-inflammatory agents affect fetal growth.

Effects mediated through inhibition of prostaglandin synthesis

All NSAIDs reduce inflammation by inhibiting prostaglandin synthesis to varying degrees. They do this by inhibiting cyclo-oxygenase (COX), an enzyme which converts arachidonic acid into prostaglandin G2. This starts a cascade releasing a multitude of prostaglandins that play a variety of biological roles. COX exists as two iso-enzymes:

- COX-1 produces prostaglandins continually to maintain the integrity of the gastric mucosa and support renal function.
- COX-2 produces pro-inflammatory prostaglandins.[15]

Currently available NSAIDs affect COX-1 and COX-2 in varying proportions. As prostaglandins play a major role in fetal development, their inhibition has various effects on the mother, fetus, and neonate (Box 7.1). Several COX-2 selective drugs will be on the market soon, e.g. Celecoxib, already licenced in the United States. These potentially reduce the gut and renal side effects but their effects on the reproductive system are not yet clear.

A retrospective study of women with musculoskeletal disorders showed that those who took more than 3.25 g of aspirin a day during the last 6 months of pregnancy had a significantly longer gestation, longer labour, and greater blood loss at delivery than women who had not taken aspirin.[16,17] Turner and Collins also found an increased incidence of anaemia, antepartum haemorrhage, and pre-eclampsia in women who took aspirin for long periods.[12] Haemostatic abnormalities and a higher incidence of intracranial haemorrhage have been found in neonates whose mothers ingested aspirin within a few days before delivery.[18,19] In the fetus, prostaglandin E causes relaxation of systemic and pulmonary vessels as well as the ductus arteriosus, and 90% of blood ejected by the right ventricle passes through the ductus arteriosus to the descending aorta.[20] In a variety of animals, administration of single doses of an anti-inflammatory agent results in reversible constriction of the ductus arteriosus and a substantial increase in pulmonary artery pressure in the fetus. Long-term exposure to anti-inflammatory agents in animals and

---

Box 7.1 Conditions associated with use of inhibitors of prostaglandin synthesis in pregnancy

- *Effects on mother:*
  - prolongation of pregnancy
  - prolongation of labour
  - increased blood loss both before and after birth
  - anaemia
  - pre-eclampsia

- *Effects on fetus and neonate:*
  - haemostatic abnormalities
  - increased incidence of intracranial haemorrhage
  - premature closure of ductus arteriosus
  - persistent pulmonary hypertension

humans is associated with increased amounts of pulmonary artery smooth muscle, which results in persistent pulmonary hypertension in the newborn infant, with or without premature closure of the ductus arteriosus.[21]

Indomethacin has been used for the treatment of preterm labour. Babies born preterm after exposure to indomethacin given for this indication have a high neonatal morbidity, with necrotizing enterocolitis, intracranial haemorrhage, and patent ductus arteriosus.[22] It is likely that the dose and duration of administration of the drug, the gestational age of the fetus at the time of exposure, and the time between the last dose of the drug and the birth of the infant are important factors. Infants born to mothers receiving long-term anti-inflammatory treatment are probably most at risk. The most potent inhibitors of prostaglandin synthesis – salicylates and indomethacin, for example – should be avoided through pregnancy and certainly during the last trimester. To minimize the effects on the fetus, drugs with a short elimination half-life and inactive metabolites – such as ibuprofen, flurbiprofen, and ketoprofen – should be used at the maximum tolerated dosage interval. More information is required about the COX-2 inhibitors before they can be prescribed in pregnancy.

The synthetic prostaglandin analogue, misoprostol, is licensed for use as a mucosal protective agent in combination with anti-inflammatory drugs. It can also be coprescribed with either naproxen (a combined pack) or diclofenac (a combined tablet). As misoprostol increases uterine tone, it should be avoided in women of childbearing age unless adequate contraception is being used.

Breastfeeding

Because NSAIDs are weak acids they do not achieve high concentrations in milk. All manufacturers state in their drug information that these drugs should not be used in lactating women. This caution is based on lack of specific information rather than known adverse reactions, and the benefit associated with breastfeeding may outweigh the risks of a carefully chosen drug. The appropriate drugs should have a short elimination half-life and metabolites which are inert or rapidly eliminated or both. Hydroxy or methyl metabolites are relatively stable in the infant's stomach, whereas glucuronide derivatives may be cleaved, releasing active metabolites.[3] Boxes 7.2 and 7.3 show the suitability of various drugs. Reported side effects are uncommon, but plasma salicylate concentrations of 1.74 mmol/litre (24 mg/dl) were found in a breastfed ound to be reversible. Many women with Wilson's disease ;iven birth to normal infants despite large doses of d-penicil- e throughout pregnancy,[43,44] and it has been proposed that in isease the fetus is protected from the effects of penicillamine e excessive maternal pool of copper. In two other surveys, ver, a ventricular septal defect was the only abnormality ted in women with rheumatoid arthritis and cystinuria.[45,46] e are about 90 case reports of penicillamine usage in preg- .[4] The evidence suggests continuing penicillamine in Wilson's e where the benefits of treatment outweigh the risks to the but discontinuing it where safer alternative drugs are ble.

astfeeding No data are available on excretion of d- illamine in breast milk. The potential toxicity makes its use dous.

munosuppressive drugs

ic agents

e antimetabolite methotrexate, a folic acid antagonist, is used increasingly to control rheumatoid and psoriatic arthri- e alkylating agents, cyclophosphamide and chlorambucil, are rarely. All three are considered teratogenic and mutagenic ven if cytotoxic agents are used after the first trimester, the is susceptible to bone marrow depression, infection, and orrhage.[47] Experience with low dose methotrexate (5 mg–20 r week) for rheumatoid arthritis is accumulating, but little en reported about its use in pregnancy. A small uncontrolled of 10 pregnancies in eight women who took methotrexate in pregnancy failed to show teratogenicity but suggested that k of spontaneous abortion may be increased.[48] No long-term s were seen in the five offspring (mean age at follow up 11.5 . Because of possible retention of methotrexate in maternal s, it is recommended that methotrexate be discontinued 2–3 s prior to conception. Folate supplementation is standard ce with methotrexate therapy. In women contemplating ancy this should be continued throughout the precon- n period and pregnancy, even when the methotrexate is tinued.

clophosphamide therapy is reserved for severe cases of vas-

Box 7.2 Suitable drugs for use during lactation

- Analgesics
  - paracetamol ⎫ See text
  - codeine ⎭

- Non-steroidal anti-inflammatory drugs:
  - ibuprofen ⎫ Small quantities in milk
  - flurbiprofen ⎪ Short elimination half-life
  - diclofenac ⎬ Inert metabolites
  - mefenamic acid ⎭

  - naproxen   Small quantities in milk
              Little ingestion by infant

  - fenoprofen ⎫ Very small quantities in milk
  - ketoprofen ⎬ Short elimination half-life
              Glucuronide metabolites not important here

  - piroxocam   Only 1–3% of maternal plasma concentra-
              tions in breast milk despite long half-life

- Disease-modifying drugs:
  - sulphasalazine   See text

- Immunosuppressive drugs:
  - Corticosteroids   See text

Box 7.3 Unsuitable drugs during lactation

- Non-steroidal anti-inflammatory drugs:
  - salicylates   Glucuronide metabolites
              Risk of Reye's syndrome

  - diflunisal ⎫
  - tolmetin   ⎬ Long half-life
  - azapropazone ⎭
  - fenbufen ⎫ Active metabolites
  - sulindac ⎭

- Disease-modifying drugs:
  - antimalarials   Risk of retinal damage
  - gold salts ⎫ Potential renal and bone marrow toxicity
  - d-penicillamine ⎭

- Immunosuppressive drugs:
  - cytotoxic agents ⎫ See text
  - cyclosporin ⎭

child with metabolic acidosis whose mother was taking 2.4 g aspirin a day, and a grand mal fit occurred in a child whose mother was taking indomethacin.[3]

Disease modifying antirheumatic drugs (DMARDs)

The drugs discussed in this section are second-line agents for the treatment of inflammatory polyarthritis, and there is a trend for starting them earlier in the course of rheumatoid arthritis to prevent joint destruction and disability. The immunosuppressive drugs are most often used for connective tissue diseases and vasculitis.

Sulphasalazine

Sulphasalazine is well established as a second-line treatment for rheumatoid arthritis. The drug reversibly reduces male sperm count but does not seem to affect female fertility. Experience of its use in the treatment of inflammatory bowel disease has shown it to be safe throughout pregnancy and lactation.[3,23,24] There is a theoretical risk of neonatal haemolysis and two case reports describe diarrhoea developing in breastfed infants.[25,26] As sulphasalazine impairs absorption of folate, supplementation is recommended in pregnancy.

Antimalarial drugs

Chloroquine salts cross the placenta and rapidly accumulate in mouse fetal tissues such as the eye.[27] Teratogenic effects are probably related to dose. Prophylactic treatment of malaria during pregnancy seems safe,[28] but exposure during the first trimester to the doses of chloroquine required to treat rheumatic diseases has been associated with sensorineural hearing loss in an infant.[29] Two studies reviewed a total of 41 pregnancies in 32 women treated with chloroquine salts:[30,31] 20 pregnancies resulted in normal babies, and the 21 fetal losses seemed to be related to disease activity rather than to treatment. In Levy's review of 215 pregnancies in women exposed to chloroquine, seven fetuses (3.3%) had congenital abnormalities.

The theoretical risk from antimalarials suggests that women should be advised to avoid pregnancy while taking chloroquine salts, but the clinical evidence shows no reason to withdraw chloro-

quine during pregnancy in rheumatoid arthritis or s erythematosus if the disease process is controlled. W reassured that pregnancy outcome is likely to be nor

Breastfeeding

Both chloroquine and hydroxychloroquine have small quantities in human milk, and the authors of dicted that an infant would be exposed to about 2% nal dose per day.[32] Despite the lack of reported adv breastfed infants of women receiving malaria prophy is advised when the drugs are used in the higher dose treating chronic rheumatic conditions. As potential r would be difficult to monitor in children of this age salts are not recommended for use in lactating wom

Gold salts

Both gold thiomalate and auranofin, an oral gol have proved teratogenic in animals.[3] Gold has been liver and kidneys of an aborted human fetus, reports of possible teratogenic effects.[33,34] Other the safe use of gold in pregnancy, and therapeutic trations have been detected in cord blood withou congenital defects.[35] Similarly, no adverse reaction 13 mothers or their infants treated with auranof pregnancy.[36] There is therefore no hard evidence to drawing treatment with gold during pregnancy if i disease. It is sensible to reduce the dose and administration.

Breastfeeding Trace amounts of gold salts have b the milk of lactating women,[37] and more recently detected in the serum of suckling infants.[38] Calc weight-adjusted dose indicated that the dose to the i that received by the mother. The theoretical possibil icity precludes its use during breastfeeding.

d-Penicillamine

The chelating agent d-penicillamine is used to tre ease, cystinuria, and rheumatoid arthritis. It cross and is potentially teratogenic. Its use in pregnancy ciated with the development of a generalized co defect similar to Ehlers–Danlos syndrome,[39–42] whic

wa
ha
lan
thi
by
hov
rep
Th
nar
dis
fett
ava

E
pen
haz

Im

Cyt

T
bei
tis;
use
and
fett
hae
mg
has
stuc
earl
the
effe
year
tissu
mor
prac
preg
cept
disc
C

culitis or life-threatening renal involvement in SLE. The risk of congenital malformation from cyclophosphamide exposure has been estimated at 16–22%.[49] The risk of infertility after treatment with cyclophosphamide increases with duration of therapy, cumulative dose and increasing maternal age.[50]

Normal pregnancy outcome has been described in increasing numbers of women taking azathioprine (a cytotoxic immunosuppressant),[51,52] although some infants have had lymphopenia, growth retardation, and an increase in chromosomal breakages. Results of a larger, longer term, follow-up study are encouraging, though mean follow-up of the children was only 6 years (range 5–13 years).[53] No increase in fetal abnormalities or abortion rate has been recorded in patients who remain fertile after cytotoxic chemotherapy. Ideally cytotoxic agents should be discontinued 2–3 months before conception is contemplated, but azathioprine may need to be continued during pregnancy to prevent a flare of the underlying disease.

Breastfeeding Cyclophosphamide and methotrexate are found in human breast milk and the potential risk to the infant precludes their use.[4] There are no data on azathioprine.

Cyclosporin

Cyclosporin is a fungal metabolite and a potent immunosuppressant. The experience of cyclosporin use during pregnancy in women who had received kidney transplants has established its safety, and case reports in other conditions (lupus nephritis, for example) are supportive.[54] It is excreted in breast milk, and the manufacturers recommend avoiding its use during lactation.

Corticosteroids

These drugs are discussed more fully in the Chapter 11. Several studies have confirmed the low risk to the fetus and mother with a rheumatic disorder of taking corticosteroids in pregnancy.[55,57] Additional doses of steroid are needed to cover delivery, but fetal adrenal insufficiency has not been described.

Breastfeeding In doses most commonly used for treating rheumatic disorders (15 mg of prednisolone or less a day) there is little chance of the infant receiving significant amounts of prednisolone in breast milk.[58]

Novel therapies in development

Leflunamide, an immunoregulator and anti-inflammatory is already licensed in the United States as a DMARD for rheumatoid arthritis. Extensive research is underway to find other potential disease-controlling drugs including monoclonal antibodies, cytokine inhibitors, adhesion molecule antagonists, gene therapy, and T-cell suppressors. The most promising so far is an antibody that blocks the effect of Tumour Necrosis Factor (TNF). Enbrel and Remicade are already available in some countries and are likely to be licensed in the UK soon. None of these agents should be used without adequate contraception until more is known about their actions.

Summary

The outlook for successful pregnancy in women with rheumatic diseases has improved in the past 10 years. With appropriate information and advice before conception, the risks to mother, fetus, and neonate can be minimized.

References

1 Office of Population Censuses and Surveys. *Morbidity statistics from general practice: third national survey.* London: HMSO, 1986.

2 Dudley DJ, Branch DW. Pregnancy in the patient with rheumatic disease: the obstetrician's perspective. In: Parke AL, ed. *Clinical rheumatology.* London: Baillière Tindall, 1990, Vol. 4, pp. 141–56.

3 Brooks PM, Needs CJ. Antirheumatic drugs in pregnancy and lactation. In: Parke AL, ed. *Clinical rheumatology.* London: Baillière Tindall, 1990, Vol. 4, 157–71.

4 Keen WF, Buchanan WW. Pregnancy and rheumatoid disease. In: Parke AL, ed. *Clinical rheumatology.* London: Baillière Tindall, 1990, Vol. 4, pp. 125–40.

5 Ramsey-Goldman R, Schulling E. Immunosuppressive drug use during pregnancy. *Rheum DisClin N Am* 1997; 23: 149–167.

6 Aviv RI, Chubb K, Lindow SW. The prevalence of maternal medication ingestion in the antenatal period. *S Afr Med J* 1993; 83: 657–60.

7 Aselton P, Jick H, Milunsky A, Hunter JR, Stergachis A. First trimester drug use and congenital disorders. *Obstet Gynaecol* 1985; 65: 451–5.

8 Bitzen PO, Gustaffson B, Jostell KG *et al.* Excretion of paracetamol in human breast milk. *Eur J Clin Pharmacol* 1981; 20: 123–5.

9 Smith G, Roberts R, Hall C, Nuki G. Reversible ovulatory failure associated with the development of luteinised unruptured follicles in women with inflammatory arthritis taking nonsteroidal anti-inflammatory drugs. *Brit J Rheumatol* 1996; 35: 458–62.

10 Collins E. Maternal and fetal effects of acetaminophen and salicylates in pregnancy. *Obstet Gynaecol* 58 (Suppl. 5): 57–62.

11 Buckfield P. Major congenital faults in newborn infants: a pilot study in New Zealand. *NZ Med J* 1973; 78: 195–204.

12 Turner G, Collins E. Fetal effects of regular salicylate ingestion in pregnancy. *Lancet* 1975; ii: 338–40.

13 Slone D, Heinonen OP, Kaufman DW, Siskind V, Monson RR, Shapiro S. Aspirin and congenital malformations. *Lancet* 1976; **i**: 1373–5.

14 Shapiro S, Monson R, Kaufman DW, Siskind V, Heinonen OP, Slone D. Perinatal mortality and birthweight in relation to aspirin taken during pregnancy. *Lancet* 1976; **i**: 1375–6.

15 Hawkey CJ. COX-2 inhibitors. *Lancet* 1999; **353**: 307–14.

16 Lewis RB, Shulman JD. Influence of acetylsalicylic acid, an inhibitor of prostaglandin synthesis, on the duration of human gestation and labour. *Lancet* 1973; **ii**: 1159–61.

17 Lee P. Anti-inflammatory therapy during pregnancy and lactation. *Clin Invest Med* 1985; **8**: 328–33.

18 Rumack CM, Guggenheim MA, Rumack BH, Peterson RG, Johnson ML, Braithwaite WR. Neonatal intracranial haemorrhage and maternal use of aspirin. *Obstet Gynaecol* 1981; **58** (Suppl. 5): 52–6.

19 Stuart MJ, Gross SJ, Elrad H, Graeber JE. Effects of acetylsalicylic-acid ingestion on maternal and neonatal hemostasis. *New Engl J Med* 1982; **307**: 909–12.

20 Rudolph AM. The effects of non-steroidal anti-inflammatory compounds on fetal circulation and pulmonary function. *Obstet Gynaecol* 1981; **58** (Suppl. 5): 63–7.

21 Levin DL, Mills LJ, Weinberg AG. Haemodynamic pulmonary vasculature and myocardial abnormalities secondary to pharmacologic constriction of fetus ductus arteriosus: a possible mechanism for persistent pulmonary hypertension and transient tricuspid insufficiency in the new born infant. *Circulation* 1979; **60**: 360–4.

22 Norton ME, Merrill J, Cooper BAB, Kuller JA, Clyman RI. Neonatal complications after the administration of indomethacin for preterm labor. *New Engl J Med* 1993; **329**: 1602–7.

23 Vender RJ, Spiro HW. Inflammatory bowel disease and pregnancy. *J Clin Gastroenterol* 1982; **4**: 231–49.

24 Newman NM, Correy JF. Possible teratogenicity of sulphasalazine. *Med J Austr* 1983; **ii**: 528–9.

25 Branski D, Kerem E, Gross-Kieselstein E, Hurvitz H, Litt R, Abrahamov A. Bloody diarrhoea – a possible complication of sulfasalazine transferred through human breast milk. *J Pediat Gastroenterol Nutr* 1986; **5**: 316–17.

26 Nelis GF. Diarrhoea due to 5–aminosalicylic acid in breast milk. *Lancet* 1989; **i**: 383.

27 Ullberg S, Lindquist N, Sjostrand S. Accumulation of chorio-retinotoxic drugs in the foetal eye. *Nature* 1970; **227**: 1257–8.

28 Lewis R, Lauersen NH, Birnbaum S. Malaria associated with pregnancy. *Obstet Gynaecol* 1973; **42**: 696–700.

29 Hart CW, Naunton RF. The ototoxicity of chloroquine phosphate. *Arch Otolaryngol* 1964; **80**: 407–12.

30 Parke AL. Anti-malarial drugs. Systemic lupus erythematosus and pregnancy. *J Rheumatol* 1988; **15**: 607–10.

31 Levy M, Buskila D, Gladman DD, Urowitz MB, Koren G. Pregnancy outcome following first trimester exposure to chloroquine. *Am J Perinatol* 1991; **8**: 174–8.

32 Nation RL, Hacket LP, Dusci LJ *et al.* Excretion of hydroxychloroquine in human milk. *Br J Clin Pharmacol* 1984; **17**: 368–9.

33 Rocker I, Henderson WJ. Transfer of gold from mother to fetus. *Lancet* 1976; **ii**: 1246.

34 Rogers JG, Anderson RMcD, Chow CW. Possible teratogenic effects of gold. *Aust Paediatr J* 1980; **16**: 195–8.

35 Cohen DL, Orzd J, Taylor A. Infants of mothers receiving gold therapy. *Arthritis Rheum* 1981; b: 104–5.

36 Ostensen M, Husby G. Antirheumatic drug treatment during pregnancy and lactation. *Scand J Rheum* 1985; **14**: 1–7.

37 Ostensen M, Skavdal K, Myklebust G *et al.* Excretion of gold in human breast milk. *Eur J Clin Pharmacol* 1986; **31**: 261.

38 Bennett PN, Humphries SJ, Osborne JP, Clarke AK, Taylor A. Use of sodium aurothiomalate during lactation. *Br J Clin Pharmacol* 1990; **29**: 777–9.

39 Mjolnerod OK, Dommerud SA, Rasmussen K, Gjeruldsen ST. Congenital connective tissue defect probably due to d-penicillamine treatment in pregnancy. *Lancet* 1971; **i**: 673–5.

40 Solomon DL, Abrahams G, Dinner M, Berman L. Neonatal abnormalities associated with d-penicillamine treatment during pregnancy. *New Engl J Med* 1977; **296**: 54–5.

41 Linares A, Zarranz JJ, Rodriguez-Alarcon J, Diaz-Perez JL. Reversible cutis laxa due to maternal d-penicillamine therapy. *Lancet* 1979; **ii**: 43.

42 Rosa FW. Teratogen update: penicillamine. *Teratology* 1986; **33**: 127–31.

43 Scheinberg IH, Sternlieb I. Pregnancy in penicillamine treated patients with Wilson's disease. *New Engl J Med* 1975; **293**: 1300–2.

44 Walshe JM. Pregnancy in Wilson's disease. *Q J Med* 1977; **46**: 73–83.

45 Lyle WH. Penicillamine in pregnancy. *Lancet* 1978; **i**: 606–7.
46 Gregory MC, Mansell MA. Pregnancy and cystinuria. *Lancet* 1983; **ii**: 1158–60.
47 Barber HRK. Fetal and neonatal effects of cytotoxic agents. *Obstet Gynaecol* 1981; **58** (Suppl. 5): 41–7.
48 Kozlowski RD, Steinbrunner JV, MacKenzie AM *et al*. Outcome of first trimester exposure to low dose methotrexate in eight patients with rheumatic disease. *Am J Med* 1990; **88**: 589–92.
49 Roubenoff R, Hoyt I, Petri M *et al*. Effects of anti-inflammatory and immunosuppressive drugs on pregnancy and fertility. *Semin Arth Rheum* 1988; **18**: 88–110.
50 Boumpas DT, Austin HA, Vaughn EM *et al*. Risk of sustained amenorrhoea in patients with systemic lupus erythematosus receiving intermittent pulse cyclophosphamide. *Ann Intern Med* 1993, **119**, 366–9.
51 Nolan GH, Sweet RL, Laros RK. Renal cadaver transplantation followed by successful pregnancies. *Obstet Gynecol* 1974; **4**: 732–9.
52 Hayslett JP, Lynn RI. Effect of pregnancy in patients with lupus nephropathy. *Kid Internat* 1980; **18**: 207–20.
53 Ramsey-Goldman R, Mientus JM, Jutzer JE, Mulvihill JJ, Medsger TA. Pregnancy outcome in women with systemic lupus erythematosus treated with immunosuppressive drugs. *J Rheumatol* 1993; **20**: 1152–7.
54 Hussein MM, Mooij JM, Roujouleh H. Cyclosporine in the treatment of lupus nephritis including two patients treated during pregnancy. *Clin Nephrol* 1993; **40**: 160–3.
55 Popert AJ. Pregnancy and adrenocortical hormones: some aspects of their interactions in rheumatic diseases. *BMJ* 1962; **i**: 967–72.
56 Yackel DB, Kempers RD, McConahey WM. Adrenocorticosteroid therapy in pregnancy. *Am J Obstet Gynecol* 1966; **96**: 985–9.
57 Grigor RR, Shervington PC, Hughes GRV *et al*. Outcome of pregnancy in systemic lupus erythematosus. *Proc R Soc Med* 1977; **70**: 99–100,
58 McKenzie SA, Selley JA, Agnew JE. Secretion of prednisolone into breast milk. *Arch Dis Child* 1975; **50**: 894–6.

8 Psychotropics

KEVIN NICHOLLS

Key points

- All women of childbearing age are potentially pregnant.
- Psychotropics in pregnancy may be indicated, but careful evaluation of risk–benefit is essential.
- Aim for the lowest effective dose.
- Polypharmacy and newer drugs should be avoided if possible, especially in the first trimester.
- Refer to secondary services at an early stage if necessary.
- Involve the mother at every stage of decision making and document fully.

Introduction

Physicians are increasingly asked for advice on prescribing psychotropic medications during pregnancy or their use in those who wish to conceive. All women of childbearing age should be considered as potentially pregnant.

Possible adverse effects of medication have to be weighed against the effects of a relapsing psychiatric disorder, including self-neglect and non-compliance with prenatal care, overdosing or other suicidal acts, and the need for more rigorous drug treatment to manage a relapsing illness compared to an alternatively stable and more benign prophylactic regimen. Some psychiatric disorders, particularly affective illnesses, are more prevalent in women over child-bearing years, and illnesses may be pharmacophysiologically different over the prenatal period. Placental function may be compromised by untreated psychiatric disorder.[1]

Approximately one-third of all pregnant women take psychotropic drugs at least once during their pregnancy.[2] The advent of antipsychotics with fewer side effects and moves towards de-institutionalization and community care, has led to an increase in fertility in women with schizophrenia and their fertility rate is now almost the same as the general population's. This group of women is more likely to suffer coerced sex and unplanned pregnancy.[3]

Three types of injurious drug effect on the embryo, fetus, or neonate are recognized:[4]

- Firstly a drug may be teratogenic. Most cross the placenta, and this includes psychotropic medications.[5]
- Secondly, neonatal withdrawal or toxicity may occur: this typically results in behavioural problems after birth. Drugs administered before birth may have prolonged postnatal effects in the new-born, owing to immature metabolism.
- Finally, longer term neurobehavioural sequelae or so-called "behavioural teratogenesis" can occur. These developmental and behavioural problems have been indicated by animal studies, and are due to effects on receptor and wider neural membrane function. Such changes in humans could result in subtle dysfunction which is difficult to detect and quantify.

Balancing relative risks against possible benefits is complicated as there is little guidance or information available, and rapid development of new drugs is a particular problem. Furthermore a change in evaluation of risk has emerged for certain drugs with consequent reassessment of previously held conventions.

The aim of this short chapter is to provide broad guidelines for sensible treatment strategies. It has to be recognized by both physician and patient that no clinical decision is totally risk-free. The outcome of consultations and jointly agreed treatment plans should always be carefully documented.

Antidepressants

Tricyclics

Tricyclic antidepressants have been available since the late 1950s. Although amitriptyline and imipramine are teratogenic in animals, over a dozen major trials have collectively looked at more than half a million births including 400 where there was first trimester exposure to tricyclics, and none have indicated excess risk.[1]

Tricyclic drugs have been implicated in perinatal syndromes, involving irritability, "jitteriness" and seizures, but reports are anecdotal and sporadic and no systematic evidence exists to suggest that this is a common occurrence.[6] No significant difference has been detected in language, intelligence quotient (IQ) or behavioural development at up to 7 years of age between tricyclic, fluoxetine, and no exposure groups; although further study of possible adverse effects on human infant development is warranted.

The evidence overall indicates that tricyclics are relatively safe, and are a treatment option in pregnancy.

Selective serotonin reuptake inhibitors (SSRIs)

Fluoxetine has been widely prescribed over the past 10 years, and most is known about this SSRI in relation to pregnancy. Animal studies have been inconclusive, some showing craniofacial abnormalities and alterations in the serotoninergic neurotransmitter systems at higher doses, whilst others have demonstrated no ill-effects.[5] Research in human populations has demonstrated rates of abnormality following exposure to fluoxetine similar to the 1–3% found in a general population. A recent prospective study of 750 women exposed to fluoxetine in the first trimester found no increase in congenital malformations, and confirmed a rate of 3%.[1]

There is some evidence that women exposed to either fluoxetine or tricyclics have a similar tendency to a higher rate of reported miscarriages. This suggests an association with the illness or other factors linked to the depressed condition. Perinatal problems described following fluoxetine include a higher rate of prematurity, increased fetal growth rate resulting in large size for gestational age, and difficulties in the neonate including CNS complications, temperature instability, irritability, tremors, and increased tone. Such problems appear to be uncommon, transient, and not dose-related.[5] All considered, there is wide consensus that fluoxetine is as safe as tricyclics in pregnancy.[7]

Other SSRIs are less well evaluated than fluoxetine. Paroxetine appears to be safe, but the evidence is limited compared to the database on fluoxetine. More recently introduced antidepressants including noradrenaline and serotonin reuptake inhibitors (NSRIs) should be avoided if possible (Box 8.1).

Guidelines for using antidepressants in pregnancy Up to 10% of women suffer from depression warranting intervention of some sort during pregnancy. Additionally there is a high rate of relapse, with as many as 50% of women who have antidepressant medication withdrawn at around conception requiring its reintroduction during the pregnancy.

On finding that she is pregnant, a woman will have to decide with her doctor whether to continue with medication. If she is taking any of the drugs in Box 8.1, a change to a traditional tricyclic or fluoxetine should be considered. Guidelines advising withdrawal of antidepressants before conception, reintrodution after the first trimester, followed by gradual withdrawal in the third trimester to avoid problems in the neonate may be too restrictive and impractical. Some women will be well into the first trimester before they recognize their pregnancy, when the potential benefit of withdrawing medication will be reduced, especially where its half-life is long. Women who prefer to come off medication should be provided

---

Box 8.1 Antidepressant drugs relatively contraindicated in pregnancy

- SSRIs
  - *paroxetine*
  - *citalopram*
  - *sertraline*

- Newer antidepressants
  - *reboxetine*
  - *venlafaxine*
  - *mirtazapine*

- Others
  - *maprotiline*
  - *mianserin*
  - monoamine oxidase inhibitors (MAOIs) including *moclobamide*

---

with psychological support, ideally by a specialist perinatal psychiatry service.

Where the woman chooses to breastfeed, the tricyclic lofepramine has theoretical advantages for nursing mothers and may be the drug chosen in pregnancy to enable continuity after delivery.[8]

Lithium

Lithium is the most widely used prophylaxis in bipolar affective disorder. Disadvantages include a narrow therapeutic index and associated toxicity. Physiological effects are complex owing to its ubiquitous distribution throughout fluid compartments and ability to displace sodium. It can, for example, affect cardiac rhythm and striated muscle function by alteration of membrane potentials. Neurotransmission and muscle contractility are also impaired through inappropriate activation of adenyl cylase. In pregnancy the lithium ion freely diffuses across the placenta, equilibrating concentration in maternal and fetal tissues.

Concerns regarding the teratogenicity of lithium led to the setting up of the Register of Lithium Babies in 1968. Initial data indicated a five-fold increase in cardiovascular abnormality following first trimester lithium, and no less than a 400–fold increase in Ebstein's anomaly (congenital incompetence of tricuspid valve with associated right ventricular defects).

However, these data are biased because lack of controls and self-reporting resulted in a slant towards cases with abnormal outcome. The excess rate of Ebstein's anomaly is now estimated as 10 to 20 times that compared to that in the general population. Since there is a baseline risk in the general population of 1:20 000 for this defect, the risk in pregnancies exposed to lithium is around 1:1000 (0.1%), translating into a small absolute risk.[6]

Other malformations reported include obstructed hydrocephalus, outer ear atresia, club feet, single umbilical artery, maxillary hypoplasia, and meningomyelocele. Isolated cases of hydramnios in the second trimester are possibly caused by lithium-induced nephrogenic diabetes insipidus.

Problems with lithium toxicity occur in the newborn at lower serum levels compared to adults, and clearance of lithium is reduced in the fetus and neonate, with a half-life as long as 96 hours. Signs of toxicity include flaccidity, cyanosis, lethargy and poor suck, and Moro-reflexes. Abnormal irritability may follow lithium withdrawal. In morphologically normal neonates, there may be an association with macrosomia, prematurity, and perinatal mortality. Transient hypothyroidism and neurological dysfunction have also been recorded.[9] Little is known about behavioural teratogenicity following lithium, but such work that has been done failed to show any effect on infant development.

Lithium treatment strategies in pregnancy

Treatment options are wider where the pregnancy is planned. If there has been only one episode of mania followed by a long period of well-being, it may be sensible to taper lithium off prior to attempting to conceive. Rapid withdrawal is associated with the risk of rebound psychosis.[10,11] Where temporary withdrawal of lithium is planned, this would necessarily include the period of 4–12 weeks post conception.

For some it might be safer to consider continuation of lithium, reducing it only after the first missed menstrual period and positive pregnancy test. This strategy minimizes the vulnerable lithium-free period, and may be of use in older women where the time taken to conceive may be longer, although more rapid lithium withdrawal is inevitable.

After stopping lithium, careful and frequent review of mental state is necessary. Empathic support, avoidance of stress where at all possible, and other psychological measures should be offered. If mood deteriorates, aggressive management at an early stage with hospitalization, reinstitution of lithium or use of other psychotropics, and consideration of electroconvulsive therapy (ECT) might minimize the overall burden of risk due to medication and illness. In some who have severe or frequent relapse of bipolar disorder, stopping lithium at any stage before, during, or after the pregnancy may be inappropriate. These women should continue with lithium subject to their informed consent following counselling. Prenatal diagnosis including expert fetal echocardiography at 16–20 weeks should be arranged if desired.

Pregnancy increases glomerular filtration rate and plasma volume, tending in turn to increase lithium clearance, and necessitating increased doses to maintain serum level. Following delivery, rapid normalization of clearance can quickly lead to toxicity, and careful monitoring is necessary at this time. The dose of lithium should be decreased by up to 50% at the onset of labour to minimize this hazard, but should not be stopped altogether, as there is increased risk of puerperal psychosis in bipolar affective disorder, which may reach over 50% depending in part on how recent the last episode of illness occurred.

Other mood disorder prophylactic agents

Substituting carbamazepine or sodium valproate for lithium in pregnancy is not recommended since these drugs are both teratogenic (see Chapter 1). Nevertheless there are no absolute contraindications, and it may be appropriate where the patient agrees to continue in a very small number of women who suffer from severe illness which may be rapid cycling, and who are not responsive to lithium,. The minimum effective dose should be used and folate prescribed. Fetal ultrasonography should be offered if appropriate between 16 and 19 weeks. Carbamazepine and sodium valproate together, or with lithium should be avoided as there may be a cumulative or synergistic risk.

Neuroleptics

The risks of not treating psychotic illness in pregnancy are serious because there may be a risk of harm to the mother or fetus, or others. Side effects of antipsychotics include hypotension, which can compromise uterine blood flow, and decreased seizure threshold. If neuroleptic malignant syndrome occurs in pregnancy, autonomic instability, dehydration, fever, renal dysfunction, and electrolyte imbalance can be exacerbated.[12]

Factors to consider when selecting a neuroleptic include the advantages of a shorter half-life and increased hydrophilicity, both of these increasing clearance from neonatal circulation.

High potency neuroleptics, including trifluoperazine and haloperidol, compare well with chlorpromazine, because they are less sedative and hypotensive; also, trifluoperazine has a half-life outer range which is half that of chlorpromazine (approximately 18 compared to 37 hours). These high potency drugs also have a "cleaner" metabolic profile than chlorpromazine, and a theoretically lower risk of teratogenicity.[13,14] Although there is a potential danger of extrapyramidal side effects in the neonate with high potency drugs, there is no evidence that this occurs. There may be a familial tendency to extrapyramidal related problems.[12] Where seizures are a special problem, a low epileptogenic drug such as sulpiride may be considered.

Teratogenicity of neuroleptics has been poorly studied scientifically. A confounding factor is the higher rate of abnormalities in children of women with schizophrenia. These pregnancies are associated with approximately the same rate of abnormality whether or not they have had chlorpromazine, yet this rate is roughly twice that of the general population.[6] Low potency neuroleptics have been most evaluated following their use for hyperemesis gravidarum in large populations of pregnant women, although in low dosages compared to the treatment of psychosis.

Haloperidol, trifluoperazine, and chlorpromazine have all been associated with congenital abnormalities, whilst individual case reports have reported limb deformities, for example. However other studies which have usually been larger but also retrospective have found no association.[6,13] Exposure to chlorpromazine between weeks 4 and 10 may be more hazardous, and phenothiazines with three-carbon aliphatic side chains (including chlorpromazine) are possibly associated with a higher rate of malformations.[6]

A metanalysis of over 74 000 births after first trimester exposure to neuroleptics has returned an odds ratio of 1.21 (although the methodology can be criticized), suggesting a statistically significant increase in relative risks. With an estimated baseline incidence of congenital abnormalities of 2%, phenothiazine use may thus increase the risk to say 2.4%, implying an additional risk of 4:1000 births (0.4%). No specific organ dysgenesis was identified.[6]

Withdrawal effects in neonates occur following *in utero* neuroleptic exposure and may be related to dopaminergic dysfunction. Animal studies indicate that exposure to neuroleptics can cause life-long depletion of dopamine receptors, and it has been suggested that developing tissue has to "see" dopamine in order to develop properly.[12]

The onset of withdrawal effects occurs between 1 and 3 days postnatally where oral medications have been prescribed, but up to 3–4 weeks' delay may occur after depot preparations. Symptoms generally resolve over a number of weeks.[12]

Problems in human neonates include increased tremulousness and restlessness, hypotonicity, and delayed motor development. Other side effects including neonatal jaundice and functional bowel obstruction; taller and/or heavier infants compared to controls have been recorded up to an age of 7 years.[12,13]

Neurobehavioural ("behavoural teratogenesis") studies have been limited, but the evidence available indicates that there is no difference in intelligence quotient (IQ) or behavioural functioning at 5 years of age.

Little information is available on the safety of the newer antipsychotic drugs. Clozapine is associated with a risk of agranulocytosis, orthostatic hypotension, and seizures. At least two case studies have been reported following exposure *in utero* to clozapine throughout pregnancy, and problems included a seizure in one infant.[15] Clozapine in common with other novel or atypical compounds are usually best avoided in pregnancy (Box 8.2).

Treatment guidelines

Acute psychosis in pregnancy is a psychiatric and obstetric emergency. Although a small proportion of women who suffer from chronic psychotic illness may improve in pregnancy, overall these women are associated with a poor fetal outcome.

Occasionally psychotic illness presents for the first time during pregnancy, and a full assessment is necessary and the need to exclude organic precipitating factors is particularly important.[6] Adequate doses of high potency neuroleptics is warranted, especially after the first trimester, the optimum dose being the lowest which controls symptoms. It may be possible to limit use of neuroleptics in these cases to an "as required" basis, or cautiously withdraw medication following resolution of symptoms.

In chronic illness the patient may be well into the first trimester by the time her pregnancy is recognized. The risk, if medication is stopped, should be appraised by review of previous illness episodes

---

Box 8.2 Atypical neuroleptics usually avoided in pregnancy

- *Risperidone*
- *Olanzapine*
- *Amisulpinide*
- *Quetiapine*
- *Clozapine*
- *Sertindole* (withdrawn as from March 1999 in UK)

---

and frequency, together with severity of relapse, especially following cessation of medication.

If the woman is on depot medication, this should usually be stopped and the commencement of oral medication delayed if possible until after the first trimester. Residues of depot over a prolonged elimination period may offer disproportionately effective protection against relapse at this time.

Where symptoms are severe or behaviour chaotic, or the risk of these is known to be high from previous history, medication may be needed on a continuing basis throughout the pregnancy. Small to moderate doses of a single drug can hold a patient in remission, comparing favourably with higher doses of several drugs which may be necessary in relapse.

If the newer antipsychotics are being prescribed, changing over to conventional high potency alternatives as soon as pregnancy is recognized should be given careful consideration (Box 8.2). However, there are no absolute contraindications, especially in cases of severe or refractory illness which has been stabilized.

Some authorities recommend the tailing off of neuroleptic medication 2 or 3 weeks prior to estimated delivery date, believing that such a strategy may reduce neonatal withdrawal symptoms, although there is little evidence that this is so. Antiparkinsonian drugs given to the mother appear to have no beneficial effects for the fetus, and may indeed compound its extrapyramidal problems. Continuing medication will usually be needed after delivery for protection during the postnatal period when the risk of relapse is high. Keeping the mother well will facilitate bonding and optimize her mothering skills. It is important to avoid oversedation during this period as this will interfere with her ability to interact with the baby.[12]

Special care is needed when the mother is breastfeeding. All neuroleptics pass into milk in appreciable quantities and although breastfeeding is not absolutely contraindicated where the dose is small, this is not recommended. It may be possible to compromise with mothers who are anxious about this by arranging a paced regimen of stored colostrum and bottle feeding.

All decisions should be jointly agreed with the patient and carefully documented. Exceptionally when illness denies the mother capacity to make decisions, compulsory admission and treatment under the provisions of the Mental Health Act may be needed. In these fortunately rare circumstances, secondary services are invariably involved, and fullest liaison with family, the obstetric team, and second-opinion doctors will be necessary.

References

1 Cohen LS, Rosenbaum JF Psychotropic drug use during pregnancy: weighing the risks. *J Clin Psychiat* 1998; **59** (Suppl. 2): 18–25.

2 Lanczik M, Knoche M, Fritze J. [Psychopharmacotherapy during pregnancy and lactation, 1: Pregnancy] [German]. *Nervenarzt* 1998; **69**: 1–9.

3 Miller LJ. Sexuality, reproduction and family planning in women with schizophrenia (Review). *Schiz Bull* 1997; **23**: 623–35.

4 Anon. Pre-conception, pregnancy and prescribing. *Drug TherBull* 1996; **34**: 25–7.

5 Baum AL, Misri S. Selective serotonin-reuptake inhibitors in pregnancy and lactation (Review). *Harvard Rev Psych* 1996; **4**: 117–25.

6 Altshuler LL, Cohen L, Szuba MP *et al.* Pharmacologic management of psychiatric illness during pregnancy: ilemmas and guidelines. *Am J Psych* 1996; **153**: 592–606.

7 Mourilhe P, Stokes PE. Risks and benefits of selective serotonin reuptake inhibitors in the treatment of depression. *Drug Safety* 1998; **18**: 57–82.

8 Nicholls KR, Cox JL. Antidepressants and breastfeeding (letter). *Psych Bull* 1996; 20: 309.

9 Goldaber KG. Psychotropics. *Sem Perinatol* 1997: **21**: 154–9.

10 Mander AJ, Loudon JB. Rapid recurrence of mania following abrupt discontinuation of lithium. *Lancet* 1988; July 2: 15– 17.

11 Margo A, McMahon P. Lithium withdrawal triggers psychosis. *Br J Psychiat* 1982; **141**: 407–10.

12 Miller LJ. Clinical strategies for the use of psychotropic drugs during pregnancy. *Psychiat Med* 1991; **9**: 275–98.

13 Pinkofsky HB. Psychosis during pregnancy: treatment considerations. *Ann Clin Psych* 1997; **9**: 175–9.

14 Cox JL, Nicholls KR. Prescibing psychotropic drugs for pregnant patients. *Prescribers' J* 1996; **36**: 192–7.

15 Stoner SC, Sommi RW,.Marken PA *et al.* Clozapine use in two full-term pregnancies (letter). *J Clin Psychiat* 1997; **58**: 364–5.

9 Epilepsy and anticonvulsant drugs

GUY SAWLE

Key points

- Enzyme-inducing anticonvulsants (carbamazepine, phenytoin, valproate, topiramate, and tiagabine) reduce the efficacy of standard dose (30 µg oestrogen) oral contraceptive pills. Higher oestrogen doses are usually necessary.

- All epileptic women of childbearing potential should receive folate supplements.

- Once a woman knows she is pregnant, the time of greatest potential teratogenic risk has probably passed.

- If a patient's epilepsy is well controlled and there are no side effects, there is little point in changing anticonvulsant during pregnancy.

- Many authorities recommend measuring anticonvulsant concentrations during pregnancy – some recommend adjusting dosage on the basis of falling concentrations, even in the absence of seizures, whilst others favour an increase only if the patient has a seizure.

- Measuring total serum concentrations gives only a crude indication of any relevant changes.

- Free valproate concentration may rise, even if the total plasma valproate concentration falls; neither correlates particularly well with seizure control.

- Because of its non-linear pharmacokinetics, there is a stronger case for measuring phenytoin concentration.

Introduction

Few situations focus the mind as well as the discovery that a patient being treated for epilepsy has become pregnant. Much of what has previously been written on this subject concerns treatment with barbiturate drugs. Outside of specialist epilepsy practice, very few women of childbearing age are now taking barbiturates, and these drugs will not be discussed further. Despite all that is written below, more than 90% of women with epilepsy have a normal pregnancy and deliver a healthy child. This chapter discusses a number of issues that commonly arise in women who are, or are intending to become, pregnant.

Contraception

Patients taking the enzyme-inducing anticonvulsants carbamazepine, phenytoin, topiramate, or tiagabine need "special" contraceptive advice, which generally means taking a higher dose pill. Usually 50 μg oestrogen is sufficient. If breakthrough bleeding occurs, contraception cannot be assured. An easy way to increase the oestrogen dose a little further is to give two 30 μg pills. Some patients need higher doses still, and it may be necessary to measure endogenous progesterone concentrations to confirm suppression of the luteal phase rise to be sure that ovulation is inhibited. Sodium valproate, lamotrigine, and gabapentin do not cause oral contraceptive failure.

Preconception folate supplements

One of the few things doctors can do that will most likely reduce the risk of fetal harm from anticonvulsants is to prescribe folate supplements in the period before conception. Folate concentrations in serum and red cells fall during pregnancy (more so in women taking anticonvulsant drugs),[1] and blood folate concentrations may have been lower in epileptic mothers who have an abnormal pregnancy outcome.[1] Neural tube defects are more common in patients taking valproate or carbamazepine (see below). Folate supplements are recommended for women who have previously given birth to a child with a neural tube defect[2] and, because of the association between anticonvulsant use and neural tube defects, it seems sensible to recommend folate supplements for all epileptic women of childbearing potential. A daily dose of 5 mg is the simplest and most convenient prescription, even though a lower dose would probably suffice. Because the timing of pregnancy is notoriously difficult to predict, the only practical way to ensure that women take folate supplements at the right time is to prescribe them immediately upon diagnosis of epilepsy during the childbearing years.

When to stop anticonvulsants

Decisions about when to stop anticonvulsants are difficult. In general, if medication is stopped after several seizure-free years, then the chance of that patient having further seizures rises to about 40% over the next few years. This sounds a high risk until it is appreciated that about 20% of a similar group of patients will have recurrent seizures over the next few years, even if they continue to take their medication. Some diagnoses, such as juvenile myoclonic epilepsy,[3] carry a particularly high risk of seizures recurring after treatment has been stopped; here the neurologist's skills in diagnosis may facilitate appropriate management. Patients whose epilepsy has been difficult to control may be at greater risk of epilepsy recurrence after stopping their medication. A decision on whether anticonvulsants should be stopped should therefore be based partly on an understanding of the epileptic diagnosis and the treatment record to date. The driving regulations may also be relevant: patients with epilepsy are usually eligible to drive once they have been free of seizures for 1 year, but are advised to stop driving for 6 months if they subsequently alter or stop their medication.

Once a woman knows she is pregnant, the time of greatest potential teratogenic risk has probably passed, so being pregnant is not really a strong reason to stop taking anticonvulsants. If the drugs are to be stopped, they should be withdrawn slowly, as they would be in a non-pregnant patient. Recommendations vary about how quickly anticonvulsants should be withdrawn. It is normally best to stop the drug in decrements over several months. In adults, each step should not exceed carbamazepine 200 mg, phenobarbitone 30 mg, phenytoin 50 mg, primidone 125 mg, and sodium valproate 200 mg.[4]

Choosing the correct anticonvulsant

There is a tradition in contemporary neurological practice to prescribe carbamazepine for patients whose seizures are of focal origin (such as in temporal lobe epilepsy), and sodium valproate for patients who have primary generalized epilepsy (such as absence seizures or juvenile myoclonic epilepsy). With few exceptions both drugs are probably equally effective for either patient group. A particular exception is juvenile myoclonic epilepsy, in which sodium valproate is the drug of choice, and carbamazepine or phenytoin may make the seizures worse.

A few years ago, carbamazepine was favoured for most women of childbearing age on the basis of a perceived lower risk of teratogenicity.[5] However, there have been reports of teratogenicity (including spina bifida) with carbamazepine, so switching almost exclusively to carbamazepine in women of childbearing potential would not now be regarded as expected practice.[6]

Some patients will be taking phenytoin. If seizures are well controlled and there are no side effects, there is little purpose in changing anticonvulsant during pregnancy, particularly as many of the putative teratogenic events will have already occurred before the mother realizes she is pregnant (for example, the palate closes by the 47th day).

Teratogenicity risks with phenytoin, carbamazepine and sodium valproate

There is an enormous literature on the teratogenic effects of anticonvulsants,[7] from which several conclusions can reasonably be drawn:

- Fetal abnormalities are more common in the children of epileptic mothers.[8] On the basis of the few published prospective studies of sufficient power to answer the question, it seems that there is about a three-fold overall increase in risk in patients with epilepsy (from about 2% in the general population to around 6% in mothers with epilepsy).[9] Most of this risk is probably due to the anticonvulsants rather than to the epilepsy itself.
- Abnormalities are more common when the mother takes more than one anticonvulsant.
- There is a particular risk of neural tube anomalies when sodium valproate is used,[10] and to a lesser extent with carbamazepine.

Retrospective versus prospective studies

Many retrospective (and uncontrolled) studies have reported high rates of malformations and anomalies in babies of epileptic mothers. Unsurprisingly, prospective studies have generally reported very much lower rates.[11] Since the background rate of fetal abnormality is of the order of 1–2%, large numbers of both epileptic and non-epileptic mothers would be needed for there to be an 80% chance of detecting a doubling of this risk at $P < 0.05$. Few prospective studies have recruited such large numbers. In a large Australian study, nine malformations were recorded amongst 244 births to epileptic mothers (3.7%), in comparison with 2099 malformations amongst 62 265 babies born to mothers without epilepsy (3.4%). This represents a relative risk of only 1.1.[12] In a large Norwegian study, 170 malformations were recorded among 3879 births to mothers with epilepsy (4.4%), compared with 136 births to 3879 mothers without epilepsy (3.5%). In this case the relative risk was 1.25.[13] In Iceland a 19–year population study of 157 women with active epilepsy revealed a 2.7 fold increase in the rate of major congenital malformations.[14] In a study with smaller numbers (119 pregnancies in mothers with epilepsy, 106 in mothers without epilepsy), the authors concluded that there was an approximate doubling of the risks of an abnormal pregnancy outcome or minor malformation. The 95% confidence intervals were 1.1–4.0 for "abnormal pregnancy outcome", and 1.0–4.0 for minor malformation.[15] These figures underscore the need to view the results of small studies with caution.

Fetal anticonvulsant syndrome

A host of congenital abnormalities has been reported in the children of mothers taking anticonvulsants, notably the "fetal hydantoin syndrome," described originally in babies born to five mothers, only one of whom was receiving phenytoin monotherapy. This "syndrome" comprises microcephaly, growth retardation, and intellectual underfunctioning, together with many less serious abnormalities, including ocular hypertelorism, distal digital hypoplasia, craniofacial, and other anomalies. Many of the dysmorphic features become less obvious as the children grow. Similar features have been reported in children of mothers treated with other anticonvulsant drugs,[16] and it has been suggested that the syndrome be renamed the fetal antiepileptic drug syndrome.

Cleft lip and palate

Cleft lip and palate are frequently cited associations with anticonvulsant drugs. A recent large case-control study reported an increase in the chance of non-syndromic cleft lip (with or without cleft palate) amounting to an odds ratio of 3.78 (95% confidence interval 1.65–7.88). In this study, both polytherapy and increased duration of epilepsy or anticonvulsant treatment increased the odds ratio. Nevertheless, in the group of patients studied (345 infants with either cleft lip or palate, 3029 unaffected infants), only 3.3% of the cleft lips and 0.9% of the cleft palates were thought to be attributable to anticonvulsant medication,[17] a reminder that congenital malformations and anomalies are common in normal pregnancy.

Spina bifida

The risk of spina bifida in children born to mothers taking valproate is of the order of 12%.[18] This is approximately the risk of recurrence in non-epileptic mothers who already have one affected child. There is also an increased risk in mothers taking carbamazepine.[19] In a meta-analysis of cohort studies published up to 1991, nine of 612 infants exposed to valproate monotherapy (1.3%) and nine of 984 exposed to carbamazepine monotherapy (0.9%) had spina bifida.[19] When data from five European studies (Berlin, Germany; Helsinki, Finland; Magdeburg, Germany; Rotterdam, The Netherlands; Institutes of Epilepsy, The Netherlands) were pooled (including 1221 children exposed to antiepileptic drugs during pregnancy), the authors found that children born to mothers taking > 1000 mg per day of sodium valproate were at considerably greater risk of major congenital abnormalities (particularly neural tube defects) than children born to mothers taking < 600 mg per day (relative risk 6.8).[20]

It is particularly important that mothers taking sodium valproate or carbamazepine have high resolution ultrasound examination at the appropriate time to detect neural tube defects. The combination of these two anticonvulsants may carry a particularly high risk in neural tube embryogenesis.

The effect of polypharmacy on teratogenic risk

Most patients with epilepsy are appropriately treated with a single agent. A minority require two or more drugs to establish and maintain satisfactory control of seizures. Women prescribed poly-therapy for epilepsy during pregnancy have a very much higher risk of fetal malformation[21,22] – an unknown part of this increased risk may be genetic, since epilepsy that is difficult to control may itself be a manifestation of an inherited disease which is likely to lead to congenital abnormalities. In a study comparing the fetal outcome of mothers taking various numbers of anticonvulsants, the malformation rate escalated from 2.4% amongst 42 infants exposed to a single agent to 7.3% in 55 infants exposed to two agents, 16.7% in 36 infants exposed to three agents, and 25% in 16 infants exposed to four agents.[22] Few patients have been fol-lowed prospectively while they have been taking particular com-binations of anticonvulsants. In one such study, seven of 12 infants born to mothers taking the combination carbamazepine plus phenobarbitone plus valproate had congenital anomalies. One possible mechanism of increased teratogenicity with poly-therapy may be that the epoxide metabolite of carbamazepine (an active and teratogenic metabolite) is less well metabolized in the presence of other anticonvulsants.[10,11]

Teratogenicity risks with lamotrigine, vigabatrin, gabapentin, topiramate, and tiagabine

There are very few data on the safety of these agents in human pregnancy. All except lamotrigine are licensed only as add-on treatments. The potential teratogenic effects of these newer agents should be discussed with women of childbearing age before these agents are prescribed.

Lamotrigine has been subjected to a wide range of mutagenicity tests in animals and the results of these tests have been interpreted to indicate that it does not present a genetic risk to humans. In the UK it has become a popular drug for use in women with epilepsy, and some neurologists consider it to be the drug treatment of choice for this group. In an observational cohort study of 11 316 patients, including 3994 who had taken lamotrigine for more than 6 months, there were no fetal abnormalities reported.[23]

Vigabatrin has been commercially available in western Europe since the end of 1989. The data sheet contraindicates the use of vigabatrin during pregnancy because of a lack of sufficient human data and an increase in cleft palate in rabbits when it is used at high doses (this may or may not be a teratogenic effect). It is known to pass across the placenta (and also into milk) in small quantities.[24]

Gabapentin has been shown to be neither genotoxic nor mutagenic by standard (animal) testing. Nevertheless, there are insufficient patient data to assess its safety during human pregnancy.

Topiramate is teratogenic in rodents (limb agenesis) and is not recommended for human use during pregnancy.

Tiagabine is not teratogenic in animals, but there are very few available data in humans.

The effect of paternal epilepsy

There is a small literature regarding the effect of paternal epilepsy on fetal well-being. Most studies have found no excess of fetal abnormality in babies born to fathers with epilepsy.[25] In a study of congenital heart defects in 2461 live-born children of parents with epilepsy, the rate of malformation was similar whether mother or father had epilepsy (1093 mothers with epilepsy, 10 heart defects; 979 fathers, eight heart defects), and the prevalence of congenital heart defects was similar to that in the background population.[26] (See also the effect of epilepsy on pregnancy below.)

Pregnancy and seizure frequency

Seizure frequency has been monitored in a small number of women with epilepsy who were not receiving anticonvulsants. In one such study of 23 pregnancies, seizure frequency increased in eight (35%).[27] Other authors reported very little, if any, significant change.[28,29] In women receiving anticonvulsants, most published data suggest that 30–50% have more seizures during pregnancy, and 10–15% have fewer seizures than during preceding months. It may be that mothers who have fairly frequent seizures (outside of pregnancy) are more likely to have an increase in frequency of seizures during pregnancy than mothers who have very infrequent attacks.[30] Sleep disturbance or deprivation during pregnancy has been held to be an important factor in changing seizure frequency, and changes in compliance and pharmacokinetics are also likely to be relevant.

Compliance with anticonvulsants during pregnancy

Most expectant mothers are wary about taking any form of drug treatment during pregnancy. Given that many will think twice before taking simple analgesia for a headache, it comes as no surprise that women with epilepsy worry about taking anticonvulsants throughout pregnancy. The risk of taking drugs is seen as a balance between benefits to the mother and harm to the unborn child (perceived as possible mayhem). Mothers may feel they are being "selfish" if they continue to take tablets to prevent the manifestations of an apparently intermittent disorder such a epilepsy. Accordingly, an unknown number of women either stop taking or reduce the dose of previously prescribed drugs. In one Japanese study, 27% were considered to be poorly compliant and suffered increased numbers of seizures.[31] In a European study 68% of the patients whose seizure frequency increased during pregnancy were reported to have been non-compliant.[27]

The effect of vomiting in pregnancy

Tablets that are vomited after being swallowed are unlikely to provide good anticonvulsant effect. It seems reasonable to suggest that patients should take a further dose if they recognize tablets in their vomit. Changing the time when tablets are taken may be helpful.

Adjusting anticonvulsant dosage in pregnancy

Even with perfect compliance, serum concentrations of anticonvulsants are liable to fall during pregnancy as a consequence of changes in circulating blood volume, protein binding, and drug clearance.[32] The ratio of free to total anticonvulsant changes, mostly in favour of an increase in the proportion of free drug. The greatest change in carbamazepine concentration occurs during the third trimester, but for other agents changes may be more pronounced earlier in pregnancy.

In some mothers, increasingly frequent seizures during pregnancy may be the consequence of pharmacokinetic change that lower cerebral concentrations of anticonvulsants, even though the dosing schedule previously controlled seizures adequately. Outside of pregnancy, patients with epilepsy who suffer further seizures are typically prescribed an increase in their anticonvulsant dose. Pregnant patients with epilepsy who have further seizures are appropriately treated in the same way. If side effects supervene after the pregnancy has finished, dosage should be decreased.

Outside of pregnancy, the best dose of an anticonvulsant is the dose that prevents seizures but does not lead to toxicity. Serum concentrations of some anticonvulsants (such as phenytoin and carbamazepine) may be used as a guide, but many (perhaps most) neurologists practising in the United Kingdom would use clinical, rather than laboratory, data to guide their prescribing.

Because of the known tendency for anticonvulsant concentrations to change in pregnancy and because of the known increase in seizures in some patients during pregnancy (but without knowledge of how many are due to changes in compliance), it has been argued that serum concentration of the drugs should be measured before (or very early during) pregnancy, and then the dose should be adjusted during the pregnancy to maintain the serum concentration that was effective previously. The relation between free and bound drug changes during pregnancy, so it would be appropriate, if using such a strategy, to measure free drug concentrations.

There is no clear evidence that such a strategy provides better control of seizures than the optimization of drug treatment on clinical grounds alone; if patients had seizures during, say, the 6 months before pregnancy, then their anticonvulsant dosage should be increased. Informed opinion is therefore divided on whether levels should be monitored with pre-emptive dosage adjustment on the basis of falling concentrations, even if the patient does not have seizures, or whether the dose should only be increased if a patient has a seizure. The Quality Standards Subcommittee of the American Academy of Neurology considers that a baseline preconception non-protein-bound anticonvulsant level, repeated at the beginning of each trimester and in the last 4 weeks of pregnancy, will be sufficient for women with good seizure control; however, note also that the primary indication for anticonvulsant dosage or drug change remains clinical, based on seizure occurrence or adverse effects.[33]

The case for measuring carbamazepine concentrations

Although there is a reasonable relation between serum carbamazepine concentrations and clinical efficacy, many practising neurologists rarely measure these concentrations in patients receiving only carbamazepine. It seems rational to measure carbamazepine concentrations during pregnancy, and this is accepted practice in a number of centres. There may be very little change in the concentration of free carbamazepine.[34] Because the absolute amount of the 10,11–epoxide (an important active metabolite) may stay unchanged,[34] and the ratio of the epoxide to total carbamazepine may increase,[9] measuring total serum concentrations may give at best a crude indication of any relevant changes.

The case for measuring valproate concentrations

The manufacturer's data sheet for sodium valproate states that "the pharmacological (or therapeutic) effects of Epilim . . . may not be clearly correlated with the total or free (unbound) plasma valproic acid level." Outside of pregnancy, most neurologists would measure valproate only in adults with suspected poor compliance (in which case a level of zero would provide useful clinical information). In pregnancy, concentrations of free valproate may rise, even if total plasma concentrations fall, so that a patient whose total plasma concentration falls may develop pregnancy-induced valproate toxicity.[35] Thus the anticipatory measurement of valproate concentrations, and particularly the practice of adjusting dosage in symptom-free patients solely because the total plasma concentration has changed, is questionable.

The case for measuring phenytoin concentrations

In a patient whose epilepsy has proved refractory to treatment with carbamazepine and valproate or who has had unacceptable side effects with those agents, treatment with phenytoin may be appropriate. The pharmacokinctics of phenytoin are notoriously non-linear, and the case for measuring drug concentrations in pregnancy is stronger than for other agents. (In fact, many of the earlier writings on the subject of seizure control during pregnancy were concerned chiefly with phenytoin.)

The effects of epilepsy on pregnancy

There have been rare reports of mothers having seizures during delivery, at a time when the fetal heart has been monitored. Generalized tonic-clonic ("grand mal") seizures may lead to profound fetal bradycardia.[9,36] Fetal cerebral haemorrhage and death has been reported after a series of seizures during pregnancy.[37] This underscores the need for good seizure control during pregnancy in the interests of fetal well-being. Rarely, (non-eclamptic) epilepsy occurs only during pregnancy and recurs with successive pregnancies. Status epilepticus is a serious complication of epilepsy; it has a mortality of about 10% outside of pregnancy and is no less serious during pregnancy – death of the child and of the mother have both been reported. It should be treated along conventional lines.[38]

The risk of spontaneous abortion is slightly increased when either the mother or the father has epilepsy. The highest risk (odds ratio 2.12) is in women with a positive family history of epilepsy.[39]

Issues surrounding delivery: use of vitamin K

Most mothers with epilepsy have a normal, uncomplicated delivery. In those taking enzyme-inducing drugs, vitamin K-dependent clotting factors may be affected. It has therefore been suggested that pregnant women taking enzyme-inducing anticonvulsants should receive vitamin K 20 mg daily for a week before delivery. Since the exact date of delivery is seldom known in advance, it seems sensible to start vitamin K, a month before the expected delivery date.[40] If this regimen is missed, the mother can be given 10 mg vitamin K parenterally during labour. Even so, fetal vitamin K concentrations will still be low, and babies born to these mothers should be given vitamin K immediately after delivery.[41]

Babies born to mothers taking benzodiazepines (or barbiturates) may suffer withdrawal symptoms after birth.

Breastfeeding

Although most anticonvulsants pass into breast milk, they do so in low concentrations and infants are likely to receive a lower daily dosage from breastfeeding than they did *in utero*. Calculations of the largest amount of drug likely to be received by a breastfed infant expressed as a percentage of the lowest recommended daily therapeutic dose for an infant are below 5% for carbamazepine and phenytoin, and under 3% for sodium valproate.[42] Lamotrigine has been measured in cord blood and the serum of an infant whose mother was treated with this drug during pregnancy and lactation, but no adverse effects were identified.[43]

What should I tell my pregnant epileptic patient?

Most of what the doctor should tell a pregnant epileptic patient should have already been covered in discussions before conception, when epilepsy is diagnosed or treated during a woman's reproductive years. Nevertheless, a number of points are worth reiterating during pregnancy.

- More than 90% of women with epilepsy have normal pregnancies and healthy infants.
- The risk of neural tube defects is increased by either sodium valproate (1–2%) or carbamazepine (0.5–1%); appropriately timed high resolution ultrasound examinations are critical.
- The newer anticonvulsants (except for topiramate) appear not to be teratogenic in animals. Human data for lamotrigine so far suggest that this is safe in human pregnancy, but there are very few data available for the other new drugs.
- Anticonvulsants that are clinically indicated should be continued throughout pregnancy; seizures during pregnancy may be dangerous; it may even be necessary to increase the dose taken during pregnancy to maintain control of seizures.
- Folate supplements should be taken throughout the reproductive years.
- Vitamin K supplements may be necessary later in pregnancy.
- Carbamazepine, sodium valproate, and phenytoin can all be taken while breastfeeding. The newer anticonvulsants are probably also safe, but there is less information available.

The prescribing physician should also carefully review the epileptic diagnosis and the need for ongoing treatment (seizure type, date of last seizure, ease of epileptic control, drug history, and driving status) may all be important here. The need for polytherapy should be carefully considered, where appropriate. If the dosage of anticonvulsants is increased during pregnancy, it may need to be reduced again during the puerperium.

References

1 Dansky LV, Andermann E, Rosenblatt D, Sherwin AL, Andermann F. Anticonvulsants, folate levels, and pregnancy outcome: a prospective study. *Ann Neurol* 1987; **21**: 176–2.
2 Anon. Folic acid to prevent neural tube defects. *DTB* 1994; **32**: 31–2.
3 Grünewald RA, Panayiotopoulos CP. Juvenile myoclonic epilepsy. *Arch Neurol* 1993; **50**: 594–8.
4 Anon. Withdrawing antiepileptic drugs. *DTB* 1989; **27**: 29–31.
5 Saunders M. Epilepsy in women of childbearing age. *BMJ* 1989; **299**: 581.
6 Chadwick D. Epilepsy in women of childbearing age. *BMJ* 1989; **299**: 1163–4.
7 Yerby MS. Teratogenicity of antiepileptic drugs. In: Pedley TA, Meldrum BS, eds. *Recent advances in epilepsy 4*. Edinburgh: Churchill Livingstone, 1988, pp. 93–107.
8 Delgado-Escueta A, Janz D. Consensus guidelines: preconception counseling, management, and care of the pregnant woman with epilepsy. *Neurology* 1992; **42** (Suppl. 5): 149–60.
9 Yerby MS. Problems and management of the pregnant woman with epilepsy. *Epilepsia* 1987; **28** (Suppl. 3): S29–S36.
10 Centers for Disease Control. Valproate: a new cause of birth defects – report from Italy and follow-up from France. i 1983; **32**: 438–9.
11 Pearse SB, Rodríguez LAG, Hartwell C, Russell G. A pregnancy register of patients receiving carbamazepine in the UK. *Pharmacoepidemiol Drug Safety* 1992; **1**: 321–5.
12 Stanley FJ, Prescott PK, Johnston R, Brooks B, Bower C. Congenital malformations in infants of mothers with diabetes and epilepsy in Western Australia, 1980–1982 *Med J Aust* 1985; **143**: 440–2.
13 Bjerkedal T. Outcome of pregnancy in women with epilepsy, Norway, 1967 to 1978: congenital malformations. In: Janz D, Dam M, Helge H, Richens A, Schmidt D, eds. *Epilepsy, pregnancy, and the child*. New York: Raven Press, 1982, pp. 289–95.
14 Olafsson E, Hallgrimsson JT, Hauser WA, Ludvigsson P, Gudmundsson G. Preganancies of women with epilepsy: a population-based study in Iceland. *Epilepsia* 1998; **39**: 887–92.
15 Steeger Theumissen RPM, Renier W, Borm CTF *et al*. Factors influencing ther isk of abnormal pregnancy outcome in epileptic women: a multicentre prospective study. *Epilepsy Res* 1994; **18**: 261–9.
16 Jones KL, Lacro RV, Johnson KA, Adams J. Pattern of malformations in the children of women treated with carbamazepine during pregnancy. *New Engl J Med* 1989; **320**: 1661–6.
17 Abrishamchian AR, Khoury MJ, Calle EE. The contribution of maternal epilepsy and its treatment to the etiology of oral clefts: a population based case-control study. *Gen Epidemiol* 1994; **11**: 343–51.
18 Lindhout D, Schmidt D. In utero exposure to valproate and neural tube defects. *Lancet* 1986; **ii**: 1142.
19 Rosa FW. Spina bifida in infants of women treated with carbamazepine during pregnancy. *New Engl J Med* 1991; **324**: 674–7.
20 Samren EB, van Duijn CM, Koch S *et al*. Maternal use of antiepileptic drugs and the risk of major congenital malformations: a joint European prospective study of human teratogenesis associated with maternal epilepsy. *Epilepsia* 1997; **38**: 981–90.
21 Lindhout D, Meinardi H, Barth PG. Hazards of fetal exposure to drug combinations. In: Janz D, Bossi L, Dam M, Helge H, Richens A, Schmidt D, eds. *Epilepsy, pregnancy, and the child*. New York: Raven Press, 1982, pp. 275–81.
22 Lindhout D, Höppener RJEA, Meinardi H. Teratogenicity of antiepileptic drug combinations with special emphasis on epoxidation (of carbamazepine). *Epilepsia* 1984; **25**: 77–83.
23 Mackay FJ, Wilton LV, Pearce GL, Freemantle SN, Mann RD. Safety of long-term lamotrigine in epilepsy. *Epilepsia* 1997; **38**: 881–6.
24 Tran A, O'Mahoney T, Rey E, Mai J, Mumford JP, Olive G. Vigabatrin: placental transfer in vivo and excretion into breast milk of the enantiomers. *Br J Clin Pharmac* 1998; **45**: 409–11.
25 Annegers JF, Hauser WA, Elveback LR, Anderson VE, Kurland LT. Seizure disorders in offspring of parents with a history of seizures – a maternal-paternal difference? *Epilepsia* 1976; **17**: 1–9.
26 Friis ML, Hauge M. Congenital heart defects in live-born children of epileptic parents. *Arch Neurol* 1985; **42**: 374–6.
27 Schmidt D, Canger R, Avanzini G *et al*. Change of seizure frequency in pregnant epileptic women. *J Neurol Neurosurg Psychiatry* 1983; **46**: 751–5.
28 Gjerde IO, Strandjord RE, Ulstein M. The course of epilepsy during pregnancy: a study of 78 cases. *Acta Neurol Scand* 1988; **78**: 198–205.
29 Tomson T, Lindbom U, Ekqvist B, Sundqvist A. Epilepsy and pregnancy: a prospective

study of seizure count in relation to free and total plasma concentration of carbamazepine and phenytoin. *Epilepsia* 1994; **35**: 122–30.

30 Knight AH, Rhind EG. Epilepsy and pregnancy: a study of 153 pregnancies in 59 patients. *Epilepsia* 1994; **16**: 1—66.

31 Otani K. Risk factors for the increased seizure frequency during pregnancy and puerperium. *Psychiat Neurolog Japon* 1985; **39**: 33–41.

32 Eadie MJ, Lander CM, Tyrer JH. Plasma drug level monitoring in pregnancy. *Clin Pharmacokinetics* 1977; **2**: 427–36.

33 Quality Standards Subcommittee of the American Academy of Neurology. Pratice parameter. Management issues for women with epilepsy (summary statement). *Neurology* 1998; **51**: 944–8.

34 Tomson T, Lindbom U, Ekqvist B, Sundqvist A. Disposition of carbamazepine and phenytoin in pregnancy. *Epilepsia* 1994; **35**: 131–5.

35 Yerby MS, Devinsky O. Epilepsy and pregnancy. In: Devinsky O, Feldmann E, Hainline B, eds. *Advances in neurology: Vol. 64. Neurological complications of pregnancy.* New York: Raven Press, 1994, pp. 45–63.

36 Teramo K, Hiilesmaa V, Bardy A, Saarikoski S. Fetal heart rate during a maternal grand mal epileptic seizure. *J Perinatal Med* 1979; **7**: 3–6.

37 Minkoff H, Scaffer RM, Delke I, Grunebaum AN. Diagnosis of intracranial haemorrhage in utero after a maternal seizure. *Obstet Gynecol* 1985; **65**: 22S–24S.

38 Shorvon S. Tonic clonic status epilepticus. *J Neurol Neurosurg Psychiatry* 1993; **56**: 125–134.

39 Schupf N, Ottman R. Reproduction among individuals with idiopathic/cryptogenic epilepsy: risk factors for spontaneous abortion. *Epilepsia* 1997; **38**: 881–6.

40 Cornelissen M, Steegers Theumissen R, Koklee L, Eshes T, Motohara K, Monvens L. Supplements of vitamin K in pregnant women receiving anticonvulsant therapy prevent neonatal vitamin K deficiency. *Am J Obstet Gynaecol* 1993; **168**: 884–8.

41 Manderbrot L, Guillaumont M, LeClerq M *et al*. Placental transfer of vitamin K1 and its implications in fetal haemostasis. *Thromb Haemost* 1988; **60**: 39–43.

42 O'Brien MD, Gilmour-White S. *Epilepsy and pregnancy. BMJ* 1993; **307**: 492–5.

43 Rambeck B, Kurlemann G, Stodieck SRG, May TW, Jurgens U. Concentrations of lamotrigine in a mother on lamotrigine treatment and her newborn child. *Eur J Clin Pharmacol* 1997; **51**: 481–4.

10 Treatment of diabetes

NICK VAUGHAN, KATE CAMPBELL

Key points

- Excellent metabolic control must be achieved before conception.

- All diabetic women who may contemplate a pregnancy should receive folic acid 5 mg daily.

- Oral hypoglycaemics are not teratogenic, but should not be used in pregnancy because they don't provide sufficiently good control for the mother and they cross the placenta.

- Tight diabetic control increases the risk of hypoglycaemia and all pregnant diabetics should carry glucagon.

Introduction

Diabetes is probably the most common disorder that influences the outcome of pregnancy. Two to three women per 1000 of reproductive age are known to have diabetes before conception, and a further significant proportion of pregnancies in otherwise normal women may be complicated by gestational diabetes. It is therefore hardly surprising that pregnancy was one of five key areas identified in the St Vincent Declaration in 1989, a statement of attainable targets for the outcomes of diabetes care, to which European government health departments are signatories. The recommendations provide the basis of an action programme for the substantial reduction of complications of diabetes.[1] For diabetes in pregnancy the objective is to "achieve pregnancy outcomes in the woman with diabetes that approximates that of the non-diabetic woman".

Pregnancy is a high-risk state for both the woman with diabetes and the fetus, and the importance of good metabolic control in pregnant women with diabetes is undisputed. Complications such as macrosomia, neonatal hypoglycaemia, miscarriage, intrauterine death, and hydramnios, as well as increased perinatal mortality rate and neonatal morbidity, can largely be prevented by intensive efforts to achieve strict normoglycaemia. A few centres now report perinatal mortality in the babies of women with insulin-dependent diabetes approaching the rate found in the normal population, but it is disappointing that this does not seem more widely achievable. It must also not be forgotten that the usual complications of pregnancy such as infection, hydramnios, pre-eclampsia, and placental insufficiency may also occur more frequently and some specific diabetic complications, particularly retinopathy, may develop or progress rapidly during gestation. Furthermore, the rate of major congenital malformations is at least two to three times higher than in non-diabetic pregnancies and this directly relates to metabolic control before and at conception.

The use of intensive home blood glucose monitoring, education concerning diabetes in pregnancy, and outpatient methods of fetal surveillance have been central to the improvement seen in the outcome of pregnancy with diabetes over recent years. Great emphasis is placed upon a multidisciplinary team approach, the team comprising diabetologist, obstetrician, diabetes nurse specialist, dietitian, neonatologist, and, most importantly, the patient herself. As a consequence, admissions to hospital have been minimized, and wherever possible uncomplicated pregnancies are allowed to go to term.

Perhaps the most important decision at this time is the choice of insulin treatment both before and during pregnancy. This must be tailored to the individual. Each patient must have an insulin regimen which provides sufficient flexibility to maintain a normal blood glucose concentration (3–6 mmol/litre) throughout the day and night, without serious hypoglycaemia, and which will also accommodate increasing insulin requirements as gestation progresses.

This chapter outlines the management of diabetes for women with established diabetes, both insulin and non-insulin dependent, and for those with gestational diabetes who require insulin therapy. It must not be forgotten that in many countries pregnant women with Type 2 diabetes substantially outnumber those with Type 1. This is a growing problem with the increasing global burden of diabetes. Some of these patients with previously unrecognized Type 2 diabetes may present during pregnancy. However, the identification of gestational diabetes is not addressed, as this is not without controversy and is well discussed elsewhere.[2,3]

Metabolic changes in normal and diabetic pregnancy

Essential to the management of diabetes in pregnancy is an understanding of the metabolic changes that occur in mothers without diabetes. Plasma glucose concentrations remain remarkably constant, although at slightly lower levels than in the non-pregnant state. This is despite increasing insulin resistance from changes in the hormonal environment, including rising levels of oestrogen, progesterone, and human placental lactogen. Enhanced insulin secretion is able to compensate for these changes but where there is inadequate functional islet-cell reserve to meet these increased insulin requirements, gestational diabetes will develop. As some 50% of patients with gestational diabetes develop non-insulin dependent diabetes later in life, it seems likely that they already have an intrinsic beta-cell defect.

Initially the metabolic adaptations of pregnancy are concerned with increased energy storage and most of the early weight gain seen in pregnancy is the consequence of fat deposition. However, the substrate demands of the fetus gradually increase and, by the end of the second trimester, these are substantial. As a result there is increasing loss of glucose to the fetus and accelerated maternal fat mobilization, leading to modestly increased plasma non-esterified fatty acid and ketone levels. This is sometimes referred to as "accelerated starvation".[4] In the patient with diabetes, this preferential transfer of glucose is particularly damaging to metabolic control in the fetus, unless there is an adequate compensatory increase in dietary carbohydrate.

The fetal beta cell is not ordinarily stimulated by physiological changes of glucose but, when maternal diabetes is poorly regulated, the fetus is exposed to much higher levels than usual. This increased metabolite delivery stimulates the fetal islet causing hyperinsulinaemia and beta-cell hyperplasia. Facilitated diffusion of glucose across the placenta becomes saturated at about 11 mmol/litre, so that the rate of transfer of glucose to the fetus does not increase when maternal blood glucose rises beyond this level.

Thus, the beneficial effects of maternal blood glucose control are only seen below about 10 mmol/litre. Improvement of control from "bad" to "average" will have little physiological effect on glucose transport and be of no benefit to fetal development and progress. Fetal hyperinsulinaemia directly leads to macrosomia, it may inhibit lung maturation and surfactant production, and enhanced beta-cell responsiveness following delivery may result in persistent hypoglycaemia.

Organization of diabetic care in pregnancy

Care should be focused in units specializing in management of pregnancy with diabetes, and is best delivered by a multidisciplinary team comprising of a diabetologist, an obstetrician with a special interest in pregnancy and diabetes, a diabetes nurse specialist, dietitian, neonatologist, and ophthalmologist. Patients should be seen frequently before, during (at least fortnightly, with telephone contact in between, until 34 weeks and then weekly), and after pregnancy. Joint clinics, with an obstetrician, diabetologist, and diabetes nurse specialist liaising closely, are the optimal arrangement. Those women developing gestational diabetes should receive the same level of care.

Preconception counselling

Pregnancies in women with diabetes should be planned. All women of child-bearing age with diabetes who envisage pregnancy should be counselled of the need for good control well before any attempts to conceive. The majority of women with Type 2 diabetes will require insulin and some preparation for this may be necessary before conception is contemplated. Congenital malformations are common in Type 2 diabetes but this probably just reflects the level of glycaemic control in early pregnancy. Despite the dramatic reductions of many of the complications related to poor metabolic control, the incidence of congenital malformations in children of mothers with diabetes remains two to three times greater than the incidence in the general population. Fatal anomalies and multiple malformations still occur more frequently than in the normal population. This has been shown to be directly related to HbA1 levels at the time of conception (Figure 10.1).[5]

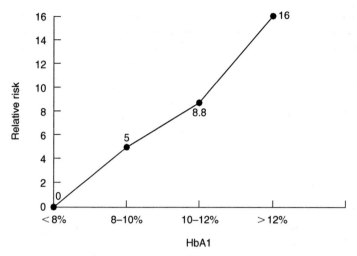

Figure 10.1   Relative risk of congenital malformation in diabetic pregnancy related to HbA1 at conception. (From Stiete *et al.*, 1994.[7])

Organogenesis for all sites in which the congenital anomalies of children of mothers with diabetes are most common is essentially complete within the first 6 weeks of gestation, before the mother may realize she is even pregnant. Pregnancy should thus ideally be deferred until prolonged good metabolic control has been attained. Evidence of this would generally be taken as a glycosylated haemoglobin in the normal range and only then should conception be sanctioned. Folate supplements should be started during this pre-conception phase and continued until the 12th week of pregnancy. In view of the association of diabetic pregnancy with spina bifida and other neural tube malformations, it seems sensible to advise women with diabetes to take 5 mg folic acid daily.[6]

Management of diabetes in pregnancy

Dietary prescription

Adequate dietary modification is perhaps the single most important aspect of management. Without this, achieving near normal glycaemic control may prove to be very difficult or impossible. Dietary prescription must meet the needs of both mother and fetus providing a total energy requirement of 30–35 kcal/kg non-pregnant ideal bodyweight. Fewer calories than this will not allow efficient protein utilization and may lead to ketogenesis induced by "accelerated starvation". It is recommended that not less than 200 g (and preferably 220–240 g) carbohydrate daily is consumed, and that this should comprise at least 50% of the total daily calorie intake,[6] as well as provide adequate fibre, calcium, and vitamins. This carbohydrate should be distributed throughout the day as regular meals and snacks, and it is especially important to provide a substantial bedtime snack (25 g carbohydrate and some protein). This helps to prevent starvation ketosis in the morning and to avoid nocturnal hypoglycaemia. Some mothers find consuming this much carbohydrate is difficult, especially if nausea is troublesome in the first trimester. However, the dietitian plays an important role in finding acceptable solutions to this, often fruit and fruit juices, and even dried fruit and nut mixtures are useful alternatives. Protein requirements increase by about 30 g a day during pregnancy, and an intake of 1.3 g/kg is generally recommended, although in practical terms many individuals already eat this much.

Women with Type 2 diabetes with normal bodyweight will need similar dietary advice to those with Type 1 diabetes. There is only a limited place for hypocaloric diets in the control of diabetes in pregnancy. However, many women with Type 2 diabetes are overweight and can tolerate a hypocaloric diet with safety, providing ketosis doesn't develop and fetal growth is satisfactory. Those who exceed 120% ideal bodyweight should be encouraged to lose weight preconception. In gestational diabetes it is usually worth attempting to correct a previously poor eating pattern, again by increasing complex carbohydrate. Good metabolic control can occasionally be achieved with such dietary measures, but such patients need careful observation with frequent checks on blood glucose and glycosylated haemoglobin values. Any suspicion of deteriorating control requires the immediate introduction of insulin and, indeed, most women with Type 2 diabetes require insulin. This would generally be indicated if the average of pre- and 2 hours postprandial blood glucose concentrations throughout the day exceeds about 6 mmol/litre.[7,8] There is probably no place for oral hypoglycaemic agents in pregnancy.

Insulin treatment

Several factors must be considered when an insulin regimen is selected. Nothing less than the attainment of normal blood glucose values throughout the day and night should be acceptable to either the patient or her physician. Any regimen must be able to take account of the substantial changes in insulin sensitivity that may increase daily doses of insulin severalfold as pregnancy progresses. Regular home blood glucose measurements are essential not only to meet the day-to-day variations in blood glucose concentrations but also to keep up with increasing insulin requirements. These should be undertaken with a home blood glucose meter with a memory (a useful check of compliance!). With this degree of surveillance and the patient's almost invariably higher motivation, it is possible to achieve sufficiently good control with most insulin regimens that entail two or more injections of a mixture of insulins. There is however a trend towards using multiple injection regimens. It is probably best if radical changes in strategy are avoided, or at least started during the period of pregnancy counselling.

Choice of insulin regimens

It is preferable to use human insulin in diabetic pregnancy, although a small minority of patients still using animal insulins, because of hypoglycaemic unawareness, may be reluctant to change. Porcine insulin is probably acceptable but bovine insulin is best avoided as it can produce significant levels of insulin antibodies that freely cross the placenta.[9] These have been implicated as a cause of infant morbidity, possibly affecting beta-cell function of the fetus and influencing neonatal insulin secretion.

Once daily insulin regimens These would seldom be appropriate in pregnant mothers with diabetes established before pregnancy, but single daily injections of an intermediate duration insulin before breakfast may be very effective in some women with Type 2 or mild gestational diabetes. Such individuals can usually produce sufficient insulin in a fasting state overnight to maintain normoglycaemia, and thus an intermediate insulin, e.g. an isophane (Humulin I [Lilly] or Insulatard [Novo-Nordisk], for example), would be suitable. Additional short-acting or soluble insulin, e.g. Actrapid (Novo-Nordisk) or Humulin S (Lilly), may be added later as a fast-acting component to counter postprandial hyperglycaemia. The use of such regimens significantly reduces the incidence of fetal macrosomia in women with gestational diabetes when compared with treatment by diet alone.[8]

Twice daily combinations of short- and intermediate-acting insulins This regimen is widely used outside pregnancy and is perfectly capable of providing adequate control during pregnancy as well.

The usual combinations are a soluble insulin with an isophane insulin. Premixed formulations of these insulins should be avoided in pregnancy as they do not afford sufficient flexibility, it is preferable to change women using these over to free-mixing their insulins during the preconception period. The ability to change the proportion of short- to intermediate-acting insulin is important because, as pregnancy progresses, the required balance between the two may change with increasing insulin resistance. Frequently, it is found that hyperglycaemia before breakfast cannot be resolved by increasing the evening dose of isophane insulin without incurring frequent hypoglycaemia during the night, partly as a result of increased transplacental passage of glucose. The general solution to this is to divide the evening injection, taking the short-acting insulin with the evening meal and the intermediate insulin at bed-time. Similarly, as gestation progresses, the proportion of short-acting insulin required may increase, reflecting increased insulin resistance; to control postprandial hyperglycaemia in the afternoon, it often becomes necessary to abandon the morning dose of intermediate insulin in preference to an additional lunch-time injection of short-acting insulin. From 36 weeks onwards, there is a tendency for the fasting blood glucose concentration to fall that may require reduction or even omission of the evening injection of intermediate insulin. Sudden dramatic falls in insulin requirements at this time should alert the clinicians to the possibility of placental insufficiency sufficient to threaten the pregnancy.

Multiple daily insulin injections   Many younger patients with diabetes already employ such regimens using pen-type insulin delivery devices. It is a particularly satisfactory means of achieving excellent metabolic control that is readily understood by the patient and can easily be altered to cope with variations in diet and activity. Generally a soluble insulin is administered with each of the main meals of the day and an isophane or insulin zinc suspension is given at bed-time. Close self-monitoring is essential for this type of regimen but this will not differ from what is required for pregnancy anyway.

Continuous subcutaneous insulin infusion (CSII)   Open loop subcutaneous insulin infusion with miniature pumps can achieve near normal glycaemic control in appropriately selected patients. However, although this was a fashionable technique a few years ago, multiple injection regimens have largely superseded pumps as very similar results can be achieved with them, and CSII is potentially more dangerous in pregnancy. Severe hypoglycaemia is a significant risk and the rapid development of ketoacidosis may occur in the event of pump failure. There is probably little place for this technique except in exceptional circumstances.

Oral hypoglycaemic agents

Commonly, women with Type 2 diabetes are taking sulphonylureas and/or metformin prior to conception. These have little place in the management of diabetes in pregnancy as glycaemic control is generally unsatisfactory. The main anxiety about sulphonylureas in pregnancy is the possibility of further increasing the degree of fetal hyperinsulinaemia by direct drug-induced stimulation. Sulphonylureas cross the placenta and have been implicated as a direct cause of neonatal hypoglycaemia.[10] The long-acting agent chlorpropamide is particularly dangerous and should not be used in the last 4 weeks of gestation. There is no convincing evidence that these drugs are teratogenic. Metformin, which does not cross the placenta, has been reported to be useful in some obese, non-insulin dependent diabetics who are inadequately controlled by diet.[11] Few would disagree, however, that judicial use of insulin is preferable.

Targets for monitoring of metabolic control

The mean diurnal blood glucose concentration in non-diabetic pregnant women is around 5 mmol/litre at 30 weeks gestation.[12] Diabetic women should be aiming at this level of control, attempting to obtain fasting and preprandial values of between 4 and 6 mmol/litre and postprandial values of less than 10 mmol/litre.[6] Home blood glucose measurement is an essential aspect of management and should be performed four to six times/day to recognize the need for insulin dose modification. This dosage adjustment can be performed by the medical team, but the patient should be encouraged and helped to gain the confidence to undertake this herself. HbA1 or HbA1c levels should be measured regularly as this provides an objective assessment of glycaemic control. Target values should be the middle of the local normal range.

Hypoglycaemia is an inevitable consequence of achieving strict glycaemic control. All women on insulin should therefore be provided with glucagon 1 mg (Lilly) or GlucaGen (Novo-Nordisk) for use in moderate to severe hypoglycaemia.

Management of labour

As regards the timing of delivery, with good glycaemic control and, in the absence of significant obstetric complications, it should be possible to prolong pregnancy until at least 39 weeks.

Dramatic changes in insulin sensitivity may occur in insulin-dependent diabetics at the time of delivery. Once active labour has started, insulin requirements fall. After delivery, once the placenta and its hormonal products have been removed, there is a further rapid reduction in insulin requirement. Indeed, immediately after delivery insulin doses may fall below prepregnancy values.

During labour the simplest scheme is to use a constant infusion of 10% glucose at a rate of 1 litre every 8 hours. An independent insulin infusion of human soluble insulin, initially at 1 unit/hour, is also given; this is subsequently adjusted on the basis of hourly bed-side blood glucose.[8] This system may be used irrespective of the last subcutaneous insulin dose but where induction or caesarean section is planned, it is best started at breakfast time after a bedtime injection of isophane insulin. As soon as the infant is delivered, the insulin infusion must be reduced or, in women with gestational diabetes, stopped altogether. The glucose infusion is continued until the next meal in patients who had vaginal deliveries or until a normal diet is resumed in those delivered by caesarean section. The prepregnancy insulin doses should resumed at this time and adjusted according to the blood sugar levels. An additional 40–50 g carbohydrate, relative to the prepregnancy dietary intake, is generally recommended during lactation. Patients should also be warned about the potential risk of hypoglycaemia whilst they are breastfeeding, especially in the middle of the night. Oral hypoglycaemic agents, where they were being used before pregnancy, are probably best avoided. Small quantities of sulphonylureas are secreted into breast milk, and therefore can theoretically induce hypoglycaemia in the infant. This is probably only of significance with the longer acting sulphonylureas such as chlorpropamide. Little is known about whether metformin is secreted into breast milk.

Although generally safe, care should be taken with the prolonged use of salt-free solutions of glucose, particularly in conjunction with oxytocin (Syntocinon) and opiates, because hyponatraemia from water retention may occur.

It has been suggested that prophylactic antibiotics should be given after operative deliveries to offset the increased risk of wound infection in women with diabetes.

Treatment of diabetic ketoacidosis

Pregnant women with diabetes are much more prone to diabetic ketoacidosis owing to the combination of insulin resistance and accelerated catabolism of pregnancy. Initiating factors are the same as for any person with diabetes and include vomiting, infections, failure of insulin administration, or failure to meet increasing insulin requirements. Ketoacidosis in pregnancy must be treated with the utmost urgency as fetal loss occurs in almost 50% of cases. Patients are best managed on a medical intensive care unit along conventional lines but with close fetal monitoring. Adequate fluid and potassium replacement is essential in conjunction with intravenous insulin infusion, adjusted to achieve a smooth reduction of plasma glucose concentration. Initial rehydration should be with normal saline; this should be changed to 10% dextrose once the blood glucose is less than 10 mmol/litre, and continued until the patient is free of ketones.

The use of corticosteroids in premature labour before 34 weeks' gestation to accelerate fetal lung maturation may dramatically increase insulin resistance. Similarly, the use of intravenous beta-sympathomimetic agents to treat premature uterine contractions will cause severe hyperglycaemia and ketoacidosis unless appropriately anticipated. Careful glucose monitoring should always accompany this form of treatment and aggressive intravenous insulin treatment must be started if necessary.

Conclusions

Remarkable improvements in the prognosis for pregnancy complicated by diabetes have been achieved in the past two decades. This has followed the recognition of the need for achieving near normoglycaemia, not only during pregnancy but also in the preconception period. The multidisciplinary team approach is central to success. The choice of insulin regimen may at first appear bewilderingly diverse, but whether there are two, three or, four injections a day, it is important only in so far as it meets the patient's individual requirements to achieve normoglycaemia safely and without serious hypoglycaemia. No regimen is ideal, much depends upon the patient's cooperation and understanding. Complex regimens are not a substitute for education and careful monitoring of diabetes.

References

1 Krans H M J, Porta M, Keen H (eds). *Diabetes care and research in Europe: the St Vincent Declaration action programme.* Genevea: WHO, 1992.
2 Naylor CD. Diagnosing gestational diabetes mellitus. is the gold standard valid? *Diab Care* 1989; **12**: 565–72.
3 Coustan DR. Gestational diabetes. *Diab Care* 1993; **16** (Suppl. 3): 8–15.
4 Freinkel N. Effects of the conceptus on maternal metabolism during pregnancy. In: Lerbal BS, Wrenshall GA (eds). *On the nature and treatment of diabetes.* Amsterdam: Excerpt Medica, 1965, p. 679.
5 American College of Obstetricians and Gynaecologists. Management of diabetes mellitus in pregnancy. *ACOG Tech Bull* 1986; No.92: 1–5.
6 Brown CJ, Dawson A, Dodds R, *et al.* Report of the Pregnancy and Neonatal Care Group. *Diab Med* 1996; **13** (9 suppl. 4): 543–53.
7 Stiete H, Stiete S, Petschaelis A *et al.* Malformations in diabetic pregnancy. *Diabetologia* 1994; **37** (Suppl. 1): A172.
8 Gillmer MD, Holmes SM, Moore MP *et al.* Diabetes in pregnancy; obstetric management. In: Sutherland HW, Stowers JM (eds). *Carbohydrate metabolism in pregnancy and the newborn.* Edinburgh: Churchill Livingstone, 1984, pp. 102–18.
9 Coustan DR, Imrah J. Prophylactic insulin treatment of gestational diabetes reduces the incidence of macrosomia, operative delivery and birth trauma. *Am J Obstet Gynecol* 1984; **150**: 836–42.
10 Adam PAJ, Schwartz R. Diagnosis and treatment: should oral hypoglycaemic agents be used in paediatric and pregnant patients. *Paediatrics* 1968; **42**: 819–23.
11 Coetzee EJ, Jackson WP. Metformin in the management of pregnant non-insulin dependent diabetes. *Diabetologia* 1979; **16**: 241–5.
12 Gillmer MD, Beard RW, Brooke FM, Oakley NW. Carbohydrate metabolism in pregnancy. Part 1. Diurnal plasma glucose profile in normal and diabetic women. *BMJ* 1975; **iii**: 402–4.

11 Treatment of asthma

CATHERINE WILLIAMSON,
CATHERINE NELSON-PIERCY

Key points

- Many asthmatic women get worse in pregnancy because they stop taking their medication.

- Regular inhaled anti-inflammatory medication is first-line maintenance treatment and is safe in pregnancy.

- The drug treatment of asthma in pregnancy is the same as in nonpregnant women.

- Steroids should be used to treat asthma in pregnancy if clinically indicated; there is no evidence that they are harmful to the fetus.

- If chest radiography is clinically indicated, then it should be performed.

Introduction

At least 3% of women of childbearing age have some degree of asthma,[1] and this prevalence is increasing in the general population and in pregnancy.[2] Asthma is by far the most common chronic illness of young adulthood, and all those involved in the care of women during pregnancy and childbirth will encounter asthmatics. This chapter outlines the normal physiological changes in the respiratory system during pregnancy and the interactions between asthma and pregnancy, and goes on to deal with the special considerations relating to prescribing for the pregnant woman with asthma.

Changes in respiratory function during pregnancy

During pregnancy, oxygen consumption is increased by around 20% and the maternal metabolic rate by about 15%. This extra demand is met by a 40–50% increase in resting minute ventilation, resulting mainly from a rise in tidal volume rather than respiratory rate. This change in ventilation may be due to the respiratory stimulant effect of progesterone. The maternal hyperventilation leads to a reduction in partial pressure of arterial carbon dioxide ($PaCO2$) to 4.0 kPa, and there is a compensatory fall in serum bicarbonate to 18–22 mmol/litre. A mild respiratory alkalosis is therefore normal in pregnancy, with an arterial pH of 7.44.

Up to three-quarters of women experience a subjective feeling of breathlessness at some time during pregnancy, possibly owing to an increased awareness of the physiological hyperventilation. This "dyspnoea of pregnancy" is most common in the third trimester and may lead to diagnostic confusion.

Late in pregnancy, the diaphragmatic elevation caused by the enlarging uterus leads to a decrease in functional residual capacity, but diaphragm excursion is unaffected so vital capacity is unchanged.

The effect of pregnancy on asthma

Published evidence about the effect of pregnancy on asthma is conflicting, and there is no consistent trend to improvement or worsening of disease severity.[3] Most studies investigating the course of asthma in pregnancy have been too small to draw valid conclusions, although a review of more than 1000 pregnant women with asthma reported in nine studies found a worsening of asthma in 22%, improvement in 29%, and no change in 49%.[4]

In general, the course of asthma in pregnancy in individual patients is unpredictable. There may be some relationship to the severity of asthma before pregnancy, in that women with only mild disease are unlikely to experience problems, whereas those with severe asthma are at greater risk of deterioration, particularly late in pregnancy.[4,5] Those women whose symptoms improve during the last trimester of pregnancy may experience postnatal deterioration.[5,6]

Whatever happens to the severity of the disease process itself, many asthmatics experience worsening of their symptoms during pregnancy simply because they have stopped or reduced their usual medication due to fears (their own or those of their doctors) about its safety.

The effect of asthma on pregnancy and its outcome

In most women, asthma has no effect upon the outcome of pregnancy. Severe, poorly controlled asthma, however, may have an adverse effect on fetal outcome.[7] This is thought to be the result of chronic or intermittent maternal hypoxaemia. Several studies have suggested a slight increase in the risk of premature labour.[7-12] These include a large prospective study from Connecticut of 3891 deliveries which found an association between maternal asthma and preterm labour (relative risk = 2.33, 95% CI = 1.03–5.26),[10] and two recent large retrospective studies.[11,12] However, two prospective case control studies of over 600 pregnancies have not confirmed these findings.[13,14] Several studies have found a higher rate of caesarean section in asthmatic pregnancies.[11-13,15] However, this may not be a result of maternal asthma, and may be a consequence of increased surveillance of asthmatic pregnancies.

There is also some evidence of an association between asthma and babies of low birthweight,[4,12,16,17] although this was not found in all studies.[13,14] Some studies have reported an increased incidence of pregnancy-induced hypertension/ pre-eclampsia in asthmatic women.[12,13,18] In over 24 000 women without essential hypertension, Lehrer and colleagues found a significant association between pregnancy-induced hypertension and asthma during pregnancy.[18] These studies need to be interpreted with caution. Women with asthma are likely to be seen more frequently during the antenatal period than normal women, and therefore to have their blood pressure measured more often. The more frequent the measurements, the more likely it is that transient increases in blood pressure will be discovered.

One study has reported an increased risk of antepartum haemorrhage and postpartum haemorrhage in asthmatic pregnancy which was independent of the treatment modality used,[2] and another found an increased risk of respiratory and urinary tract infection.[19] However, these findings have not been reported in other studies.

Some studies suggest a possible increased incidence of transient tachypnoea of the newborn (TTN),[20] neonatal hypoglycaemia,[13] neonatal seizures,[21] and admission to the neonatal intensive care unit[11] in the babies of asthmatic women, but the magnitude of effect on any adverse perinatal outcome is certainly small and related to the degree of control of the asthma.

One retrospective study reported a higher incidence of congenital abnormalities in the children of asthmatic women,[12] but this has not been shown to occur in two large prospective studies of over 650 pregnancies in asthmatic women,[13,14] nor in one subsequent retrospective case control study of 101 pregnancies.[19]

In conclusion, it seems that there may be a slight increased risk to the babies of asthmatic mothers, but this risk is small and may be minimized by maintaining good control of asthma throughout pregnancy.

Management of asthma in pregnancy

Much unnecessary impairment of quality of life results from failure to diagnose or adequately treat asthma. Since virtually all women are under some form of medical supervision during pregnancy, this is an ideal time to recognize previously undiagnosed asthma and to achieve optimum disease control in women known to be asthmatic.[22]

The successful management of asthma during pregnancy requires a cooperative approach between the obstetrician, the physician managing the asthma, and the woman. The aim of treatment is to achieve virtual total freedom from symptoms, such that the life-style of the individual is not affected. The past 10–15 years have seen major changes in approaches to asthma management. The emphasis now is on the prevention, rather than the treatment, of acute attacks. Regular inhaled anti-inflammatory medication is now considered first-line maintenance treatment for all but those with infrequent symptoms (less than once a day).[23] If this does not control a woman's symptoms, high dose inhaled steroids, or the long-acting inhaled beta-agonist, salmeterol, are recommended.[23] If this is not sufficient, either a theophylline, inhaled ipratropium, or a course of regular steroid tablets can be tried.

There is also now a greater focus on home peak flow monitoring and personalized self-management plans, which have been shown to reduce morbidity in asthmatics.[24,25] Peak flow meters can be prescribed to help women to monitor their asthma throughout pregnancy.

Drug treatment

The drug treatment of asthma in pregnancy is, in essence, no different from the treatment of asthma in non-pregnant women. All the drugs in widespread use to treat asthma, including systemic steroids seem to be safe (Table 11.1). Considerations concerning individual treatments are discussed below. Table 11.2 summarizes the major studies of the pregnancy outcome of women who were taking specific drugs to treat asthma in pregnancy. Only studies with a control group are included.

Corticosteroids Systemic corticosteroids have serious and well-known side effects when given frequently or in high doses for prolonged periods. Women and their doctors are accordingly reluctant to use these drugs in pregnancy, and their concern extends to the use of inhaled corticosteroids. This concern is misplaced, and

Table 11.1 The safety of drugs which can be used for the treatment of asthma in pregnancy

Drug	1st Trimester	2nd Trimester	3rd Trimester
Inhaled/ nedulized beta$_2$-agonists	Safe	Safe	Safe
Inhaled corticosteroids	Safe	Safe	Safe
Oral corticosteroids	Safe	Safe	Fetus: Safe Maternal effects: ↑ risk of impaired glucose tolerance; pre-eclampsia; adrenal insufficiency
Inhaled salmeterol	Safe	Safe	Safe
Theophyllines	Safe	Safe	↑ risk of neonatal jaundice; otherwise safe
Inhaled cromoglycate	Safe	Safe	Safe
Anticholinergics	Safe	Safe	Safe
Leukotriene antagonists	Unsure	Unsure	Unsure

Table 11.2 Complications of asthma medication in pregnancy

Drug	No. of cases	Congenital malformations	Other adverse outcomes	Reference
Inhaled bronchodilators	259	Not increased[a]	Not increased[a]	37
	470	Not increased[a]	Not increased[a]	28
Inhaled corticosteroids	45	Not increased[b]	Possible increased LBW[b]	34
	2014	Not increased[b]	Not reported	35
	89	Not increased[a]	Not increased[a]	28
Oral corticosteroids	261	Not increased[b]	Not increased[b]	29
	58	Not reported	Increased pre-eclampsia[a]	13
	31	Not increased[a]	Increased LBW, prematurity and maternal impaired glucose tolerance[a]	11
Inhaled salmeterol	93	Not increased[b]	Not reported	28
Theophyllines	212	Not increased[a]	Increased pre-eclampsia and neonatal jaundice[a]	44
	429	Not increased[a]	Not increased[a]	28
Cromoglycate	243	Not increased[a]	Not increased[a]	28

This Table (modified from Schatz[28]) summarizes the major studies in which the pregnancy outcome in women who were taking specific drugs for asthma was compared with that of controls. [a] Compared with an unexposed control group; [b] Compared with the general population; LBW = low birthweight.

steroids should be used to treat asthma in pregnancy in the same way and for the same reasons as outside pregnancy.

Short courses of oral steroids are required for exacerbations of asthma that fail to respond to an increased dose of inhaled steroids, and for acute severe attacks. Rarely, a patient with severe asthma may require long-term maintenance oral steroids. Such individuals will always also take inhaled steroids to minimize the oral dose requirement and risk of the usual systemic steroid side effects.

Other than media-fed concern about drugs falling within the broad category of "steroids", there is a single 40–year-old report of an increased incidence of cleft palate in the offspring of rabbits treated with cortisone early in gestation.[26] This finding has never been reproduced in humans despite the fact that steroids have been used extensively during pregnancy for a variety of conditions. Prednisolone is metabolized by the placenta and very little (10%) active drug ever reaches the fetus. There is no evidence of increased risk of abortion, stillbirth, congenital malformations, adverse fetal effects, or neonatal death attributable to treating the asthmatic mother with steroids.[8,9,27–29]

A recent prospective observational study was performed to compare the birth size and subsequent development of 477 preterm infants whose mothers were given either single or repeated antenatal doses of betamethasone to prevent respiratory distress syndrome. Repeated courses of this corticosteroid resulted in significant reductions in birthweight and head circumference.[30] The authors expressed concern that the reduced head circumference may impair the subsequent intellectual development of infants who receive repeated doses of corticosteroids antenatally. However, there are no prospective studies to establish whether this is a problem at present. In addition, it is important to remember that betamethasone crosses the placenta more readily than prednisolone, the corticosteroid used to treat asthma in pregnancy, of which only 10% of the active drug reaches the fetus.

Although suppression of the fetal hypothalamic-pituitary–adrenal axis is a theoretical possibility when the mother is treated with systemic steroids, there is no evidence from clinical practice to support this. Further reassurance comes from a study in which the adrenocortical reserve of six newborns whose mothers had received long-term systemic steroids was formally assessed – the response to exogenous adrenocorticotrophic hormone was normal.[31] Maternal adrenal insufficiency is, however, a possibility, and if the woman has been taking more than 7.5 mg of prednisolone for 2 weeks or more, parenteral steroids (hydrocortisone 100 mg three or four times a day) should be given to cover the stress of labour and delivery.

Prolonged use of oral steroids increases the risk of gestational diabetes, and causes a deterioration in blood glucose control in those women with established impairment of glucose tolerance in pregnancy. Provided clinicians are aware of this and check the blood glucose regularly, the hyperglycaemia is amenable to treatment with diet and, if required, insulin, and is reversible the steroid dose is stopped or reduced. The development of hyperglycaemia is not however an indication to discontinue or decrease the dose of oral steroids, the requirement for which must be determined by the asthma.

Two studies have reported an increased risk of pregnancy-induced hypertension in oral corticosteroid treated asthmatics.[2,15] In addition, a large study of 1044 asthmatic and 860 control pregnancies demonstrated an increased risk of pre-eclampsia in 130 patients who had taken oral corticosteroids (odds ratio 2.0, $P = 0.027$).[28] However, the authors concluded that, given the maternal and fetal consequences which may result from severe asthma, the use of oral corticosteroids remains clinically indicated in the treatment of asthma in pregnancy.

The rare, but important, psychiatric side effects of oral glucocorticoids should be remembered, and all women who have been commenced on steroids should be reviewed within 1 week.

Few women with asthma will be taking oral steroids; most will be receiving inhaled steroids. As with systemic steroids, no harm to the fetus from inhaled steroids has been shown. Furthermore, only minimal amounts of inhaled corticosteroid preparations are systemically absorbed.[32] This should be emphasized, as decreasing or stopping treatment with inhaled anti-inflammatory drugs during pregnancy often causes potentially dangerous deterioration in disease control.

Beclomethasone dipropionate is the oldest inhaled steroid preparation, and therefore the drug for which most information exists. Several studies have shown no increased incidence of congenital malformations or adverse fetal effects attributable to the use of inhaled beclomethasone in pregnancy.[9,33,34] In addition, a large study of the more recently introduced inhaled steroid budesonide revealed no increase in the incidence of congenital malformation in the 2014 infants studied.[35] Use of a spacer device when inhaled steroids need to be administered will reduce oropharyngeal candidiasis, improve delivery of the drug, and decrease the possibility of systemic effects.

Fluticasone propionate is a newer inhaled corticosteroid. There are no published reports of maternal or fetal hazards, and although the drug has been available for several years, the manufacturers are not aware of any adverse events (personal communication). However, it is sensible to use a more long-established alternative if possible.

In summary, inhaled, nebulized, oral, and parenteral corticosteroids are safe in pregnancy. The addition of systemic corticosteroids to control exacerbations of asthma is appropriate, and these must not be withheld if current medications are inadequate.

Beta$_2$-agonists Inhaled beta$_2$-agonists such as salbutamol and terbutaline provide rapid and effective relief of bronchospasm in most patients. Tremor and tachycardia are the most common dose-related side effects of these drugs, but they occur far less commonly than with the now little used oral preparations. Maternal pulmonary oedema, hypokalaemia, and hyperglycaemia are potential but rare adverse effects when high doses of beta$_2$-agonists are given intravenously (to treat acute severe asthma or preterm labour).

Transfer of beta$_2$-agonists from the systemic circulation across the placenta is relatively rapid,[36] but very little of a given inhaled dose reaches the lungs, and only a minute fraction of this reaches the systemic circulation. Two prospective studies of over 700 pregnant asthmatics treated with inhaled beta$_2$-agonists showed no difference in perinatal mortality, congenital malformations, birthweight, Apgar scores, or delivery complications when compared with asthmatics not using beta$_2$-agonists and non-asthmatic controls.[28,37] Because of their proven tocolytic effect in preterm labour, there has been concern that beta$_2$-agonists may delay the onset of labour or prolong its duration, but there is no evidence that this occurs with inhaled preparations. A study of 130 pregnant asthmatics who were treated with oral beta$_2$-agonists revealed no increase in congenital malformations.[37]

The inhaled long-acting beta$_2$-agonist, salmeterol, may be used in some patients who have not achieved adequate control of symptoms with regular inhaled corticosteroids and short-acting drugs. Salmeterol is especially useful for those with nocturnal asthma.[38] A UK prescription event monitoring study which included 93 pregnant asthmatics who had been treated with salmeterol found no increase in the rate of congenital malformations.[39] One baby was born with faciodigitogenital syndrome, but several members of the family also suffered from the condition. There have been no other studies of the use of salmeterol in pregnancy, and although there is less information regarding safety than for older treatments, we would not recommend discontinuing its use in pregnant asthmatics.

Disodium cromoglycate and nedocromil Inhaled cromoglycate is generally more widely used in the management of asthma in children than in adults. It seems to be safe for both mother and fetus. A French study of nearly 300 pregnant women showed no increased risk of malformations.[40] This was confirmed in an American study of 243 women,[28] and there have been no suggestions of other ill effects in over 30 years of use.

Nedocromil is a more recently introduced preparation with a pharmacological action similar to sodium cromoglycate.

Methylxanthines These drugs are no longer used as first-line therapy for asthma. A modified-release oral preparation may be added to conventional therapy with inhaled bronchodilators and inhaled corticosteroids, especially to control night-time symptoms and early morning wheeze. Both theophylline and aminophylline readily cross the placenta and fetal theophylline levels are similar to those of the mother.[41] Although theophylline has been shown to be a potent cardiovascular teratogen in animals, there is no conclusive evidence of ill effect or malformation in the human fetus.[23,42–44] One recent prospective study of 429 women who took theophylline in pregnancy (292 in the first trimester) and 1061 controls demonstrated no increased risk of major congenital malformation (4.7% of theophylline treated women vs 5.3% of controls).[28] There is just one report linking theophylline with congenital cardiac anomalies in the human.[45] One study of 212 theophylline treated asthmatics, 292 pregnant asthmatics without theophylline, and 237 controls demonstrated double the frequency of neonatal jaundice necessitating treatment, but this may be explained by a trend to more prematurity in the theophylline treated group.[44]

Pharmacokinetic data concerning xanthines in pregnancy are conflicting. The increased blood volume associated with pregnancy may lead to lower concentrations of active drug. In contrast, a small study suggested a 20–35% reduction of theophylline clearance in the third trimester,[46] but this has not been confirmed by more recent studies.[40,47,48] Some have noted transient tachycardia or irritability in neonates of mothers receiving xanthines, but others found mean neonatal heart rate and Apgar scores were unaffected by maternal use of theophylline.[41]

Anticholinergic drugs Anticholinergic drugs have traditionally been considered more effective in the management of chronic bronchitis than asthma, but inhaled ipratropium bromide may be worth trying when symptoms are not optimally controlled with regular inhaled corticosteroids and beta$_2$-agonists. No adverse fetal affects have been reported but, as with atropine, there is a minimal increase in fetal heart rate.

Leukotriene antagonists Leukotrienes are metabolites of arachidonic acid which act as mediators of inflammation, and cause smooth muscle constriction and proliferation. Leukotriene antagonists have been recently introduced, and can be taken orally. Montelucast is currently licenced in the UK as monotherapy for the prophylaxis of exercise-induced asthma in patients aged 6 years and over. Zafirlucast is licensed in patients over 12 years of age, and can be used as first-line therapy instead of inhaled corticosteroids. At present there is insufficient information to establish whether the leukotriene antagonists are safe in pregnancy. However, the manufacturer is aware of 73 pregnancies which have occurred while women were taking zafirlucast to treat asthma (personal communication with the authors). In the 43 where they were aware of the outcome, there were 24 normal babies, 10 terminations, 8 miscarriages, and one baby was born with a heart murmur which was not believed to be due to the zafirlucast treatment.

Management of acute severe asthma

Acute severe attacks of asthma are dangerous and should be vigorously managed in hospital. There were three deaths from asthma in the UK during the period 1994–1996,[49] two of these occurring post partum. The treatment is no different from the emergency management of acute severe asthma in the non-pregnant patient. Oxygen, nebulized bronchodilators, oral or intravenous steroids, and, in severe cases, intravenous aminophylline or intravenous beta$_2$-agonists should be used as indicated. Sudden severe deterioration, or failure to respond to treatment should raise the possibility of a pneumothorax. The ionizing radiation from a chest X-ray is approximately 0.2 rad (less than 1/20th of the maximum ided exposure in pregnancy [5 rad]), and abdominal shielding will minimize the exposure to the fetus. If a chest X-ray is clinically indicated this investigation must not be withheld just because the patient is pregnant.

Other considerations when prescribing for the pregnant asthmatic

Education and reassurance of asthmatic women before conception as well as during pregnancy are integral parts of management. This should ensure that women do not discontinue, reduce, or withold vital medication just because they are pregnant. Women with asthma may justifiably be reassured about the outlook for themselves and their baby during pregnancy.

Aspirin

Low dose aspirin is used as prophylaxis for certain women at very high risk of early onset pre-eclampsia,[50] but it is worth remembering that some asthmatics are allergic to aspirin. The prevalence of aspirin sensitivity in pregnant asthmatics was 15% in a study of 504 women.[44] Therefore it is important to ask about a history of such sensitivity before treatment is started with low dose aspirin.

Management of respiratory infection

Upper and lower respiratory tract infections, bacterial and viral, are common precipitants for deterioration in asthma. The production of yellow or green sputum is not pathognomonic of a lower respiratory tract infection, and may just indicate an exacerbation of asthma with eosinophils in the sputum. However, if there are other pointers to infection (e.g. fever, chest signs), antibiotics should be prescribed.

The antibiotics most frequently used in respiratory infections, including the penicillins, cephalosporins, and erythromycin, are safe in pregnancy. Amoxycillin should be given in higher than usual dosage (500 mg 8-hourly) in pregnancy because of increased renal clearance. Tetracycline causes permanent staining of the child's teeth, has adverse effects on the fetal skeleton, and is contraindicated in pregnancy, with rare exceptions where the health of the mother takes precedence over the risk to the fetus. Similarly, cough medicines containing iodine are contraindicated since the iodine is taken up by the fetal thyroid and may cause hypothyroidism and fetal goitre.

Adults in general and pregnant women in particular are susceptible to varicella zoster (chickenpox) pneumonia, and the maternal and fetal mortality is high.[51] Because of the substantial risk to the mother, non-immune pregnant women exposed to varicella should be given zoster-immune globulin.[52] Patients taking systemic corticosteroids are at especially high risk of severe varicella, and it has been suggested that patients should be asked about a previous history of varicella prior to commencing steroids.[53] If the history is doubtful, antibody status should be checked and those who are found to be seronegative must be told to attend immediately and receive prophylaxis with zoster-immune globulin following inadvertent exposure to varicella.

Management during labour and delivery

Although they are one of the most common fears of asthmatic women entering pregnancy, acute attacks of asthma during labour and delivery are extremely rare, and women should be reassured accordingly. The explanation for this rarity is uncertain, although it is possible that it is related to an increase in endogenous corticosteroid or catecholamine production at this time. None of the three maternal deaths from asthma referred to above occurred during labour.[49] Women should continue their regular inhalers throughout labour, and those on maintenance oral steroids (> 7.5 mg prednisolone daily), or being treated with steroids for more than 2 weeks before the onset of labour or delivery, should receive parenteral steroids during labour, and until they are able to restart their oral medication. Prostaglandin E_2 used to induce labour, to ripen the cervix, or for early termination of pregnancy is a bronchodilator and is safe to use. Prostaglandin $F_{2\alpha}$, carboprost, used in the emergency management of postpartum haemorrhage, may cause bronchospasm, especially in conjunction with general anaesthesia.[54,55]

All forms of pain relief in labour, including epidural analgesia and Entonox, may be safely used by asthmatic women, although opiates should be avoided, in the unlikely event of an acute asthmatic attack. If anaesthesia is required, women should be encouraged to have epidural rather than general anaesthesia because of the increased risk of chest infection and associated atelectasis in people with asthma. Although ergometrine has been reported to cause bronchospasm, particularly in association with general anaesthesia, this does not seem to be a practical problem when Syntometrine (oxytocin + ergometrine) is used to prevent post-partum haemorrhage.

NSAIDs are commonly used for pain relief post-caesarean section. Women with asthma should be asked about any known aspirin, or NSAID, allergy prior to the use of these drugs. If a woman has such a history, it is safer to use an alternative form of analgesia.

Breastfeeding

Women with asthma should be encouraged to breastfeed their babies if they wish. The risk of atopic disease developing in the child of an asthmatic woman is about one in 10, or one in three if both parents are atopic. There is some evidence that this risk may be reduced by breastfeeding. A 15-year prospective study has shown that breastfeeding and delaying exposure to allergens reduces the frequency of clinical allergic disease,[56] and prolonged breastfeeding may lower the incidence of severe or obvious atopic disease particularly in babies with a family history of atopy.[57]

All the drugs employed in the management of asthma, including oral steroids, are safe to use when breastfeeding. Small amounts of prednisone and prednisolone are secreted in breast milk,[58,59] and, although continuous maternal use of high doses of corticosteroids could theoretically affect the infant"s adrenal function, this is unlikely with doses below 30 mg prednisolone per day. No clinical side effects have been reported in infants breastfed by mothers receiving prednisolone. A small study examining the secretion of tritium-labelled prednisolone in breast milk showed a mean of only 0.14% of radioactivity from an oral dose of 5 mg of prednisolone was recovered per litre of breast milk.[59]

Theophylline appears in breast milk, with a milk to plasma ratio of 0.7, reaching a peak concentration 2 hours after peak plasma levels.[60] We are not aware of any reports of significant problems in clinical practice resulting from transfer of methylxanthines in breast milk, and the proportion of new mothers who need methylxanthines is in any case extremely small.

Conclusion

Management of asthma in pregnancy does not differ significantly from management outside pregnancy. The priority should be effective control of the disease process, with the aim being total freedom from symptoms both day and night. Great attention must, however, be given to explanation and reassurance about the safety, in pregnancy and during lactation, of the drugs used to treat asthma.

The small risk of harm to the fetus comes from poorly controlled severe asthma rather than from the drugs used to prevent or treat asthma. Good control of asthma reduces the already small risks of preterm delivery or low birthweight. Furthermore, it sets a pattern for future management; the mother–infant relationship may not flourish in the presence of chronic maternal ill health. Asthma in pregnancy should accordingly be regarded as an opportunity to gain long-term benefit, not just as a challenge lasting nine months.

Acknowledgements

The authors would like to acknowledge Dr John Moore-Gillon, an author of this chapter in the second edition of this book, for his substantial contribution.

References

1 Littlejohn PI, Ebrahim S, Anderson R. Prevalence and diagnosis of chronic respiratory symptoms in adults. *BMJ* 1989; **298**: 1556–60.
2 Alexander S, Dodds L, Armson BA. Perinatal outcomes in women with asthma during pregnancy. *Obstet Gynecol* 1998; **92**: 435–40.
3 Sims CD, Chamberlain GVP, de Swiet M. Lung function tests in bronchial asthma during and after pregnancy. *Br J Obstet Gynaecol* 1976; **83**: 434–7.
4 Gluck JC, Gluck P. The effects of pregnancy on asthma: a prospective study. *Ann Allergy* 1976; **37**: 164–8.
5 White RJ, Coutts I, Gibbs CJ, MacIntyre C. A prospective study of asthma during pregnancy and the puerperium. *Respir Med* 1989; **83**: 103–6.
6 Juniper EF, Daniel EE, Roberts RS, Kline PA, Hargreave FE, Newhouse MT. Improvement in airway responsiveness and asthma severity during pregnancy. A prospective study. *Am Rev Resp Dis* 1989; **140**: 924–31.
7 Bahna SL, Bjerkedal T. The course and outcome of pregnancy in women with bronchial asthma. *Acta Allergolog* 1972; **27**: 397–400.
8 Schatz M, Patterson R, Zeitz S, O"Rourke J, Melam H. Corticosteroid therapy for the pregnant asthmatic patient. *JAMA* 1975; **233**: 804–7.
9 Fitzsimons R, Greenberger PA, Patterson R. Outcome of pregnancy in women requiring corticosteroids for severe asthma. *J Allergy Clin Immunol* 1986; **78**: 349–53.
10 Doucette JT, Bracken MB. Possible role of asthma in the risk of preterm labor and delivery. *Epidemiology* 1993; **4**: 143–50.
11 Perlow JH, Montgomery D, Morgan MA, Towers CV, Porto M. Severity of asthma and perinatal outcome. *Am J Obstet Gynecol* 1992; **167**: 963–67.
12 Demissie K, Breckenridge MB, Rhoads GG. Infant and maternal outcomes in the pregnancies of asthmatic women. *Am J Respir Crit Care Med* 1998; **158**: 1091–5.
13 Stenius-Aarniala B, Piirila P, Teramo K. Asthma and pregnancy: a prospective study of 198 pregnancies. *Thorax* 1988; **B**: 12–18.

14 Schatz M, Zeiger RS, Hoffman CP et al. Perinatal outcomes in the pregnancies of asthmatic women: a prospective controlled analysis. *Am J Respir Crit Care Med* 1995; **151**: 1170–4.
15 Wendel PJ, Ramin SM, Barnett-Hamm C, Rowe TF, Cunningham FG. Asthma treatment in pregnancy: a randomized controlled study. *Am J Obstet Gynecol* 1996; **175**: 150–4.
16 Greenberger PA, Patterson R. The outcome of pregnancy complicated by severe asthma. *Allergy Proc* 1988; **9**: 539–43.
17 Schatz M, Zeiger RS, Hoffman CP. Intrauterine growth is related to gestational pulmonary function in pregnant asthmatic women. Kaiser-Permanente asthma and pregnancy study group. *Chest* 1990; **98**: 389–92.
18 Lehrer S, Stone J, Lapinski R et al. Association between pregnancy-induced hypertension and asthma. *Am J Obstet Gynecol* 1993; **168**: 1463–6.
19 Minerbi-Codish I, Fraser D, Avnun L, Glezerman M, Heimer D. Influence of asthma in pregnancy on labor and the newborn. *Respiration* 1998; **65**: 130–5.
20 Schatz M, Zeiger RS, Hoffman CP, Saunders BS, Harden KM, Forsythe AB. Increased transient tachypnoea of the newborn in infants of asthmatic mothers. *Am J Dis Child* 1991; **145**: 156–8.
21 Patterson CA, Graves WL, Bugg G, Sasso SC, Brann AW Jr. Antenatal and intrapartum factors associated with the occurrence of seizures in term infant. *Obstet Gynecol* 1989; **74**: 361–5.
22 Moore-Gillon JC. Asthma in pregnancy. *Contemp Rev Obstet Gynaecol* 1993; **5**: 25–9.
23 The British Guidelines on Asthma Management: 1995 review and position statement. *Thorax* 1997; **52** (Suppl.): S1–21.
24 Beasley R, Cushley M, Holgate ST. A self-management plan in the treatment of adult asthma. *Thorax* 1989; **44**: 200–4.
25 Charlton I, Charlton G, Broomfield J, Mullee MA. Evaluation of peakflow and symptom only self management plans for control of asthma in general practice. *BMJ* 1990; **301**: 1355–9.
26 Fainstat T. Cortisone-induced congenital cleft palate in rabbits. *Endocrinology* 1954; **55**: 502.
27 Snyder RD, Snyder D. Corticosteroids for asthma during pregnancy. *Ann Allergy* 1978; **41**: 340–1.
28 Schatz M, Zeiger RS, Harden K, Hoffman CP, Chilingar L, Petitti D. The safety of asthma and allergy medications during pregnancy. *J Allergy Clin Immunol* 1997; **100**: 301–6.
29 Schatz M, Hoffman CP, Falkoff R *et al*. The course and management of asthma and allergic diseases during pregnancy. In: Middleton E, Reed CE, Ellis EF, Adkinson NF, Yunginger JW, eds. *Allergy: principles and practice*, 3rd edn. St Louis: CV Mosby; 1988, pp. 1124–5.
30 French NP, Hagan R, Evans SF, Godfrey M, Newnham JP. Repeated antenatal corticosteroids: Size at birth and subsequent development. *Am J Obstet Gynecol* 1999; **180**: 114–21.
31 Arad I, Landau H. Adrenocortical reserve of neonates born of long-term, steroid-treated mothers. *Eur J Pediatr* 1984; **142**: 279–80.
32 Harris DM. Some properties of beclomethasone dipropionate and related steroids in man. *Postgrad Med J* 1975; B: 20–5.
33 Marion-Brown H, Storey G. Beclomethasone dipropionate aerosol in long-term treatment of perennial and seasonal asthma in children and adults. A report of five and a half-years experience in 600 asthmatic patients. *Br J Clin Pharmacol* 1977; **4**: 529s–67s.
34 Greenberger P, Patterson R. Beclomethasone dipropionate for severe asthma during pregnancy. *Ann Intern Med* 1983; **98**: 478–80.
35 Kallen B, Rydhstroem H, Aberg A. Congenital malformations after the use of inhaled budesonide in early pregnancy. *Obstet Gynecol* 1999; **93**: 392–5.
36 Morgan DJ. Clinical pharmacokinetics of beta-agonists. *Clin Pharmacokinet* 1990; **18**: 270–94.
37 Schatz M, Zeiger RS, Harden KM et al. The safety of inhaled beta-agonist bronchodilators during pregnancy. *J Allergy Clin Immunol* 1988; **82**: 686–95.
38 Fitzpatrick MF, Mackay T, Driver H, Douglas NJ. Salmeterol in nocturnal asthma: a double blind, placebo-controlled trial of a long acting inhaled beta2-agonist. *BMJ* 1990; **301**: 1365–8.
39 Mann RD, Kubota K, Pearce G, Wilton L. Salmeterol: a study by prescription event monitoring in a UK cohort of 15,407 patients. *J Clin Epidemiol* 1996; **49**: 247–50.
40 Wilson J. Utilisation du cromoglycate de sodium au cours de la grossesse. *Acta Ther* 1982; **8**: 45–51.
41 Labovitz E, Spector S. Parental theophylline transfer in pregnant asthmatics. *JAMA* 1982; **247**: 786–8.

42 Greenberger P, Patterson R. Safety of therapy for allergic symptoms during pregnancy. *Ann Intern Med* 1978; **89**: 234–7.

43 Heinonen DP, Stone D, Shapiro S. *Birth defects and drugs in pregnancy*. Littleton, Mass: Publishing Sciences Group, 1977.

44 Stenius-Aarniala B, Riikonen S, Teramo K. Slow-release theophylline in pregnant asthmatics. *Chest* 1995; **107**: 642–7.

45 Park JM, Schmer V, Myers TL. Cardiovascular anomalies associated with prenatal exposure to theophylline. *South Med J* 1990; **83**: 1487–8.

46 Carter BL, Driscoll CF, Smith GD. Theophylline clearance during pregnancy. *Obstet Gynaecol* 1986; **88**: 146–9.

47 Frederikson MC, Ruo TI, Chow MJ et al. Theophylline pharmacokinetics in pregnancy. *Clin Pharmacol Ther* 1986; **40**: 321–8.

48 Gardner MJ, Schatz M, Cousins L et al. Longitudinal effects of pregnancy on the pharmacokinetics of theophylline. *Eur J Clin Pharmacol* 1987; **31**: 289–95.

49 Department of Health, Welsh Office, Scottish Home and Health Department and Department of Health and Social Services, Northern Ireland. *Confidential enquiries into maternal deaths in the United Kingdom 1994–96*. London: HMSO, 1998.

50 CLASP (Collaborative low-dose aspirin study in pregnancy) Collaborative Group. CLASP: a randomized trial of low-dose aspirin for the prevention and treatment of pre-eclampsia among 9364 pregnant women. *Lancet* 1994; **343**: 616–29.

51 Broussard RC, Payne DK, George RB. Treatment with acyclovir of varicella pneumonia during pregnancy. *Chest* 1991; **99**: 1045–7.

52 Parayani SG, Arvin AM. Intrauterine infection with varicella-zoster virus after maternal varicella. *New Engl J Med* 1986; **314**: 1542–6.

53 Rice P, Simmons K, Carr R, Banatvala J. Near fatal chickenpox during prednisolone treatment. *BMJ* 1994; **309**: 1069–70.

54 Fishburne JI Jr, Brenner WE, Braaksma JT, Hendricks CH. Bronchospasm complicating intravenous prostaglandin F2@a for therapeutic abortion. *Obstet Gynecol* 1972; **39**: 892–6.

55 Hyman AL, Spannhake EW, Kadowitz QJ. Prostaglandins and the lung: State of the art. *Am Rev Respir Dis* 1978; **117**: 111–36.

56 Gruskay FL. Comparison of breast, cow, and soy feedings in the prevention of onset of allergic disease: a 15–year prospective study. *Clin Pediatr Phil* 1982; **21**: 486–91.

57 Saarinen UM, Kajosaari M, Backman A, Siimes MA. Prolonged breast-feeding as prophylaxis for atopic disease. *Lancet* 1979; **ii**: 163–6.

58 McKenzie SA, Selley JA, Agnew JE. Secretion of prednisolone into breast milk. *Arch Dis Child* 1975; **50**: 894–6.

59 Katz FH, Duncan BR. Entry of prednisone into human milk. *New Engl J Med* 1975; **293**: 1154.

60 Yurchek AM, Jusko WJ. Theophylline secretion into breast milk. *Pediatrics* 1976; **57**: 518.

12 Drugs of abuse

MARY HEPBURN

Key points

- Amenorrhoea is common among heroin users but conceptions can still occur.

- Naloxone can precipitate severe antepartum fetal distress in heroin and methadone users.

- Breastfeeding can minimize neonatal withdrawal in heroin and methadone users.

- Breastfeeding is not advisable in benzodiazepine users.

Introduction

Problem drug use among women of childbearing age has increased by almost 500% in the past 20 years[1] so drug use by pregnant women is seen with increasing frequency. Patterns change with time and vary from area to area, with polydrug use being increasingly common. Use of cannabis is widespread throughout the UK and is not confined to those who have a drug problem. In England in 1995 amongst those seeking treatment for drug problems[2] 80% of female users were aged 15–34 years. Opiate/opioid use was most common, reported as the main or subsidiary drug by more than 90% of those attending (64% heroin, 30% methadone and 6% "other opiates") and as the main drug of use by more than two-thirds. Amphetamines were next most commonly reported, but this nevertheless represents an underestimate of use. Benzodiazepines as main drug of choice were less common, but awareness of illicit benzodiazepine use, particularly with opiates/opioids, has been steadily increasing.[3,4]

In Scotland opiate/opioid use is similarly most commonly reported,[5] with heroin followed by methadone as the main drug. of use. Use of benzodiazepines by injection is a major problem in Scotland and particularly Glasgow[6], with injection in combination with opiates/opioids considered an important factor in drug deaths. A third of those seeking help are women of whom over 90% are aged 15–34 years. Overall in the UK more than a third of those seeking treatment were currently injecting their drugs. The route of use has obvious implications for the severity of effects on pregnancy.

Problem drug use occurs more frequently in association with socioeconomic deprivation and the poorer pregnancy outcomes are multifactorial. Identifying the precise effects of the drug use quantitatively or qualitatively can therefore be difficult.

Conception

Heroin has been claimed to cause increased levels of circulating gonadotrophins with an increased incidence of multiple pregnancies,[7] but more commonly it is reported to cause reduced gonadotrophin production, secondary amenorrhoea[8,9] and consequently infertility. While amenorrhoea is common among heroin users it is important to be aware that this may occur with or without anovulation, so for those who do not want to conceive adequate contraception is essential.

Use in pregnancy

General effects on mother and baby

The drugs most commonly used illicitly fall broadly into three main categories:

- sedative or depressant (opiates, opioids, benzodiazepines, cannabis)
- stimulant (amphetamines, cocaine)
- perception altering or hallucinogenic (LSD, high dose cannabis).

Drug misuse is illegal and self-reporting of drug use is often unreliable. In addition, patterns and levels of use are not constant and polydrug use is common even in the presence of prescribed substitute medication. Many reported data derive from relatively small samples so, for all these reasons reliable data on effects of drug use on pregnancy outcome are difficult to obtain.

There have been inconsistent reports of increased congenital abnormalities but no good evidence of teratogenesis from the drugs most commonly used illicitly. Significant misuse of drugs in pregnancy is associated with higher rates of perinatal mortality and morbidity but this is only partly due to the effect of the drugs, with a major contribution from social problems either predisposing to or a consequence of drug use. Low birthweight is the most frequently observed adverse outcome owing to reduced fetal growth and/or preterm delivery, while increased rates of sudden infant death are reported. These outcomes are all increased in the presence of socioeconomic deprivation and associated factors such as cigarette smoking. Neonatal withdrawal symptoms from opiate/opioid and/or benzodiazepine use often pose the biggest management challenge as well as causing considerable maternal distress.

Sedative drugs

Opiates/opioids **Heroin**. Opiates and opioids are the most commonly misused drugs of which heroin is the most frequently reported by those seeking help for addiction problems. Heroin obtained illicitly is in a brown powder containing various other substances which can themselves be harmful. It is commonly smoked in cigarette form or heated over tin foil and inhaled ("chasing the dragon") or injected. There is no evidence of teratogenesis, but heroin causes reduced fetal growth.[10] Its use in pregnancy is associated with increased perinatal mortality and morbidity, attributable largely to increased rates of low birthweight from intrauterine growth retardation with or without preterm delivery.[11,12] An increased risk of sudden infant death syndrome (SIDS) is also reported[13] thought to be related to the observation of reduced fetal breathing and reduced fetal response to carbon dioxide[14].

Heroin has a relatively short half-life, so many of the adverse effects are caused or exaggerated by repeated minor degrees of withdrawal. Withdrawal causes smooth muscle spasm; uterine contractions may precipitate preterm delivery or abortion (although the latter is difficult to quantify), whilst placental vasoconstriction may cause fetal compromise and reduced intrauterine growth. Spasm of the fetal gut may lead to antepartum passage of meconium. Major degrees of rapid withdrawal may cause acute fetal stress, as suggested by the observation of increased levels of amniotic fluid catecholamines following acute maternal withdrawal of opiates[15]. For this reason it has been widely held that antenatal detoxification is dangerous and should only be undertaken in mid-trimester, if at all, and then only at very slow rates. However, experience in Glasgow has demonstrated that, in practice, despite the theoretical risks, detoxification at any speed and at any stage of pregnancy is not unacceptably hazardous to the fetus[16]. However, the same cannot be said of reversal with naloxone which may precipitate severe antepartum fetal distress or shock in the neonate and should be used only with extreme caution. Planned rapid detoxification should be carried out under obstetric supervision and should, of course, only be undertaken if it is the woman's choice. Rapid detoxification is justified when substitute prescribing is not available, but, even if it is undertaken by choice, it carries a significant risk of relapse. During pregnancy it is therefore usually preferable to prescribe substitute medication in the form of methadone with either steady dose maintenance or subsequent reduction in dosage or detoxification from methadone as appropriate. Other substitute drugs are available but are either unevaluated or contraindicated in pregnancy.

Heroin causes withdrawal symptoms in the neonate, with timing of onset and severity depending on pattern and level of maternal use. If it is used up to the time of delivery, symptoms usually appear within 24 hours, increasing over the next day or two and resolving within a week. The severity of symptoms is largely dose dependent but can be increased by intrapartum fetal asphyxia, and decreased by prematurity with immaturity of the neurological system.

Other opiates/opioids, such as dihydrocodeine, and other types of drugs, especially benzodiazepines, also cause neonatal withdrawal, so unexpectedly severe or prolonged symptoms may reflect poly-drug use. Maternal dosage therefore cannot be used accurately to predict the likelihood or severity of withdrawal, nor can the baby's condition be taken to reflect the mother's level of use accurately.

Heroin is present in breast milk. However, this means that breastfeeding can be helpful in avoiding or minimizing withdrawal symptoms in the baby and, in the absence of contraindications, should be advocated, provided that drug use is reasonably stable. In addition, breastfeeding should not be suddenly discontinued, since this might precipitate withdrawal symptoms in the baby.

Contraindications would include maternal HIV infection. The significance of maternal HCV infection is less certain but, given the lack of evidence of transmission of HCV infection by breastfeeding and the enormous benefits of breastfeeding (in addition to reduction of withdrawal symptoms) for this group of vulnerable babies, many would consider it justifiable to recommend breastfeeding.

The question of what constitutes stability of drug use is widely debated. However, since breastfeeding requires application and effort in practical terms the successful establishment of breastfeeding is in itself an adequate demonstration of sufficient stability of drug use. Moreover, once they have succeeded in establishing breastfeeding, few women stop suddenly, although it is important to ensure that they know the dangers of doing so. In the absence of a major contraindication, such as maternal HIV infection, it is therefore reasonable to advocate at least an attempt at breastfeeding by all women using opiate/opioid drugs.

Information about long-term effects of drug use on child development is difficult to obtain because of difficulties in maintaining contact, and difficult to interpret because of confounding factors. It has been reported that maternal heroin use in pregnancy is associated with ongoing growth impairment with behavioural disturbances,[17] but genetic, antenatal, and postnatal environmental factors may be significant. Long-term outcome is reported to be better among women maintained on methadone,[18] but this may reflect the fact that, compared to women using heroin, women on methadone usually have greater stability of drug use, as well as other aspects of lifestyle, with more regular attendance for antenatal care.

Methadone. Methadone is an opioid available as tablet, linctus, or injectable liquid, and is the most commonly prescribed substitution drug for those dependent on opiates and opioids. It is socially beneficial because it removes the need to finance drug use by crime, stabilizes lifestyle, and brings users into contact with support services. Medically it is preferable to heroin because, in addition to being legal, it is pure, is usually prescribed in the oral linctus form and, of particular benefit in pregnancy, it has a long half-life with a duration of action in excess of 24 hours. This eliminates the fluctuations in blood levels of drug which occur with heroin use and which are harmful to the fetus.

The appropriate dose is the lowest compatible with stability but the decision as to whether to reduce the dose should be agreed with each woman on an individual basis, and the amount or rate of any reduction should be dictated by her wishes and her ability to cope. It should be remembered, however, that methadone as an opioid shares many effects with the drug(s) it replaces and, as the dose increases, the cost/benefit balance will shift.

Methadone is associated with reduced birthweight,[18] which becomes more significant as the dose increases. Like heroin, it is reported to increase the risk of SIDS,[19] and reduced fetal breathing and response to carbon dioxide are observed.[14] It is often advised that it is necessary to increase the dose of methadone in late pregnancy, but in practice this is not the case and, indeed, women often achieve their most significant reductions in dosage, as impending delivery with the prospect of neonatal withdrawal symptoms strengthens their motivation. At this stage it is important to ensure that their goals are realistic and to emphasize the importance of stability rather than abstinence. It is also important to remember that such reductions achieved in the short term may not be sustainable in the long term, and it may be necessary to increase the methadone dose postnatally to ensure ongoing stability. Objectives in substitute prescribing may therefore be rather different in pregnancy.

Some would argue that substitution therapy with methadone is not justified for non-injecting use of heroin or other opiates/opioids such as dihydrocodeine. However, removal of the cost of illicit drug use, often necessitating illegal activities, together with stabilization of lifestyle and contact with services, is sufficient justification; also, in pregnancy the longer action of methadone and consequent benefit for the fetus will justify substitution therapy in more marginal situations than might otherwise be the case. While the greatest increase in perinatal mortality is reported to occur with continued use of heroin on top of prescribed methadone, this refers to significant use of both drugs, and is probably attributable to instability of lifestyle and associated factors,[20] rather than direct effects of the drugs per se; unlimited increases in methadone dosage in (sometimes futile) pursuit of total abstinence from all illicit drugs may therefore be less beneficial to the fetus than very occasional use of non-injected heroin on top of a more modest dose of methadone when this is associated with stability of lifestyle. In pregnancy there may therefore be a lower threshold for prescribing methadone but a more conservative approach to dosage.

Methadone also causes withdrawal symptoms in the neonate later than with heroin. They are often apparent within 48 hours and are usually obvious by 3–5 days of age, resolving within 10 days or so but occasionally lasting longer. Again severity is largely dose-dependent, but is influenced by other perinatal factors; unexpectedly severe or prolonged symptoms may indicate polydrug use, especially when this involves benzodiazepine use.

Methadone is also present in breast milk and the arguments already given in favour of breastfeeding by women using opiates/opioids apply here. For women stable on long-term maintenance methadone, the question of how long to continue breast-feeding is often raised. Whilst prolonged breastfeeding especially in the presence of a high dose of methadone might not be desirable, there is no obvious endpoint, and decisions should be individually made; however, for all women on methadone it would be reasonable to continue for at least 6 months or so, to achieve maximum benefits for the baby.

The problems of assessing long-term effects of methadone use on child development are similar to those for use of heroin. However, it seems likely from the limited data available that maternal methadone therapy per se is not detrimental,[18] and adverse environmental factors are probably of greater significance.[21]

Buprenorphine. This is a partial opiate agonist available as a sublingual tablet or injectable liquid. It is marketed as a mild/moderate analgesic but, contrary to initial claims, has addictive properties, and is therefore misused. The sublingual tablets are highly soluble and therefore injectable. In Scotland in the 1980s, buprenorphine was extensively misused at doses many times the recommended therapeutic range and was the foremost drug of choice among those addicted to opiates/opioids. At dosages associated with misuse, it has effects similar to those of heroin, with increased rates of low birthweight from growth retardation and/or preterm delivery. Buprenorphine has recently been used as substitute medication, mainly in detoxification, on the grounds that it is claimed to be easier to withdraw from than methadone. Trials of use of buprenorphine in pregnancy are underway with claims that it causes less severe neonatal withdrawals than methadone, but as yet there are no trial data on its efficacy or safety in pregnancy. However, data relating to its illicit use in pregnancy by several hundred women in Glasgow, although uncontrolled, suggest outcomes were no worse than with methadone; whilst the amounts used illicitly were many times greater than recommended therapeutic doses, they were still much lower than those recommended for treatment of drug misuse.

Buprenorphine also causes neonatal withdrawal symptoms which are similar in timing to those due to heroin.

Again, buprenorphine is present in breast milk and, in the absence of contraindications, breastfeeding should be advocated.

Dihydrocodeine. Marketed as an analgesic for moderate pain, dihydrocodeine is available in oral and injectable forms. The latter is a controlled drug, but the oral form is not and is consequently sometimes prescribed as opiate/opioid substitution by doctors reluctant to prescribe methadone. At doses associated with misuse it has effects similar to heroin with increased rates of low birthweight from retarded fetal growth and/or preterm labour. Meconium staining of the liquor is also more frequently observed. Whilst these effects may be related to dihydrocodeine's short duration of action, anecdotal evidence suggests they may be disproportionately pronounced.

Dihydrocodeine causes neonatal withdrawal symptoms that are usually apparent within 24 hours. These symptoms may be severe and prolonged, and overall severity again often appears out of proportion with the level of drug use. Some women top up their methadone with oral dihydrocodeine in the belief that the latter does not constitute "drug use", and this may be a factor when methadone withdrawals seem unexpectedly severe or prolonged. These observations are purely anecdotal but controlled scientific data are difficult to obtain and these effects are observed with sufficient frequency to justify advising against use of dihydrocodeine in pregnancy.

Dihydrocodeine is present in breast milk but the adverse effects on the fetus, including severe withdrawal symptoms in the baby, make the risk/benefit ratio less clear, and efforts during pregnancy and after delivery, especially if the woman is breastfeeding, should be directed towards cessation of use or substitution by another less harmful drug such as methadone.

Other opiates/opioids. A variety of other drugs are misused, including morphine (various preparations), dipipanone (Diconal), pethidine, dextromoramide (Palfium), pentazocine (Fortral), dextropropoxyphene (with paracetamol as Distalgesic or co-proxamol), and various codeine-containing analgesics. In general they cause symptoms similar to those described for the more common opiates/opioids, although there may be both quantitative and qualitative differences. Many of the analgesics prescribed for mild/moderate pain will therefore adversely affect the fetus if used alone, and will also contribute to and exacerbate neonatal withdrawal symptoms if they are used in combination with other opiates/opioids. Their use should therefore be borne in mind if a baby becomes ill with symptoms strongly suggestive of drug withdrawal, or if the baby of a known user develops unexpectedly severe withdrawal symptoms. The possibility of misuse should always be borne in mind when such analgesics are being prescribed, especially if they are requested on a recurrent basis; their potentially harmful effects on the fetus should also be remembered when they are prescribed to women who may become pregnant.

Benzodiazepines Legal prescription of benzodiazepines peaked around 1980 but, as this has diminished, illicit use of a wide range of preparations has increased, particularly among young people. They are used illicitly both orally and by injection, with temazepam particularly liable to be injected. They are used in association with cocaine to reduce the depressant effects which follow its use and, together with opiates/opioids, to increase the pleasurable effects. As already discussed, benzodiazepine use in combination with other drugs, especially opiates/opioids, is increasingly common, and use by injection of temazepam together with heroin is a major problem in Scotland.[6] The doses of benzodiazepines used are often very high, and women who also use benzodiazepines are in all respects very unstable compared to women who use opiates/opioids alone.[3]

Claims that there is an increased incidence of cleft palate associated with benzodiazepine use have not been substantiated.[22] Associations with pyloric stenosis, cardiac defects, inguinal hernias, and craniofacial defects have also been reported.[23,24] However, in Glasgow among several hundred women who used benzodiazepines at all stages of pregnancy, often in association with opiates/opioids, often by injection, and in more than 90% of cases in combination with smoking, no such association has been observed (Hepburn, unpublished data). Growth retardation as reported in one small study[24] has been observed, but in the presence of variable polydrug use and instability of lifestyle, the precise contribution from benzodiazepine use per se is difficult to quantify.

Benzodiazepines cause withdrawal symptoms in the baby that are often evident in the first 24–48 hours, especially with shorter acting drugs such as temazepam, and can be very troublesome and often prolonged. They are often very similar to those caused by opiates/opioids and, where the drugs are used in combination, it may be difficult to distinguish effects from each type; the net effect is of severe and prolonged withdrawals. This effect is often heightened by the adverse effects of benzodiazepine use on the mothers' parenting skills.

There is no evidence that substitution therapy reduces the level of use or improves stability of drug use or lifestyle, so management should be directed towards maternal withdrawal. If this is sudden, it may precipitate convulsions in the mother. However, regardless of level of use, complete withdrawal can be safely achieved within a week with the use of a longer acting drug, such as diazepam (which is also an effective anticonvulsant), with an initial level as low as 30–40 mg/day in divided doses and daily reduction of one dose in rotation. There should be no attempt to reduce levels of opiate/opioid use during withdrawal from benzodiazepines. Relapse is not uncommon and repeated attempts at benzodiazepine withdrawal may be necessary. This is not an indication that it should not have been attempted in the first place, since any reduction in use, even if not sustained in the long term, will be of benefit to the fetus. It is also important to remember that subsequent overenthusiastic or unrealistic reduction in methadone dosage may precipitate resumption of top-up use of benzodiazepines.

The benzodiazepines that are commonly used illicitly pass into the breast milk and, because of the effects on both mother and baby, breastfeeding is unlikely to be successful and is not advisable.

Stimulants

Amphetamines Amphetamine (alpha-methylphenethylamine) can be swallowed, snorted, smoked, or injected. Illicitly obtained amphetamine is highly impure with only a small amount of amphetamine mixed with a variety of other substances, some of which may have harmful effects. There are no specific effects associated with amphetamine use in pregnancy, and with intermittent or recreational use no evidence of effect on pregnancy outcome. With high continuous levels of use, growth retardation may occur, but unstable lifestyle with poor nutrition will be contributory factors. In high dosage and especially by injection, amphetamine use is more harmful; for example, consequences reported by the Edinburgh Poisons Bureau include bleeding disorders and abdominal pain, a combination which may suggest placental abruption. Such a presentation is, however, very rare. At common levels of use, short-term increases in pulse and blood pressure have little effect, but in all cases the clinical picture may be confused by effects of substances used to cut the amphetamines or by drugs used in combination with it.

There is debate about the role of substitution therapy for amphetamine users. Its use is sometimes justified for heavy and/or injecting users on the grounds that it may bring them into contact with support services and reduce levels of injecting. However, its role in the management of pregnant amphetamine users is less clear, and many would consider the potential benefits insufficient to justify its use in this setting.

Amphetamines do not cause withdrawal symptoms in the baby, and breastfeeding, in the absence of contraindications, should be encouraged.

Ecstasy Ecstasy use is largely recreational; it does not lead to significant physical dependence and, even at high levels, is not usually associated with the instability of lifestyle and consequent problems seen with use of opiates/opioids or benzodiazepines. There is no evidence of adverse effects on pregnancy nor of withdrawal symptoms in the baby, and breastfeeding is not contraindicated.

Cocaine Cocaine is available as cocaine hydrochloride and as crack cocaine, the latter produced by heating cocaine hydrochloride with sodium bicarbonate. Cocaine hydrochloride illicitly obtained is impure and the powder is either sniffed/snorted or injected, and is sometimes injected in combination with heroin (speedball). Crack cocaine is pure crystalline cocaine which is usually smoked, but can be injected if first made soluble by mixing with an acid such as vitamin C. Use of cocaine by snorting is commonly recreational but injected cocaine and crack by any route are associated with dependent use, and polydrug use is common. There is no suitable or effective substitution therapy for cocaine, so many users do not present to services but, increasingly, pregnant women with drug problems may report use of cocaine along with other drugs.

The difficulties in identifying and quantifying specific drug effects on pregnancy outcome and factors which influence reporting have been well illustrated in the case of cocaine. Cocaine is widely regarded as a particularly harmful drug if used in pregnancy. There are numerous reports of adverse outcomes including congenital malformations,[25] spontaneous abortion,[26] placental abruption,[26,27] growth retardation,[28,29] preterm delivery,[28,30] and sudden infant death syndrome.[31] Cocaine is a powerful vasoconstrictor, and vascular compromise has been suggested as a common aetiology for many fetal abnormalities, including limb reduction defects and non-duodenal intestinal atresia, symmetrical growth retardation, spontaneous abortion, and placental abruption.[32] Such findings are inconsistent with other reports of no increase in congenital malformations or preterm delivery.[29] It is widely acknowledged that the nature and/or extent of adverse outcomes is difficult to determine because of the frequent presence of other factors such as low socioeconomic status and associated problems. However, there is good evidence of a bias against publication of studies which do not report adverse outcomes.[33] There is no doubt that heavy uncontrolled use of cocaine together with an unstable and unhealthy lifestyle will increase the risk of adverse pregnancy outcomes; it seems likely that lesser recreational use does not have similar effects.

Cocaine does not cause neonatal withdrawal symptoms. Problems in the baby, if they occur, are attributable to antenatal complications. Breastfeeding is not invariably contraindicated in the presence of any cocaine use; decisions about breastfeeding should be made individually on the basis of presence or absence of contraindications and stability of lifestyle.

Hallucinogenic drugs

LSD Use of LSD in pregnancy is usually intermittent and recreational. No specific problems have been demonstrated in association with its use in pregnancy and it does not cause withdrawal symptoms in the neonate. Substitution therapy is neither available nor necessary.

Cannabis Cannabis use is widespread in the UK and therefore relatively common among pregnant women. It can be taken orally but is usually smoked either on its own or together with tobacco. The individual contributions of cannabis and tobacco to observed outcomes are difficult to determine but it has been reported to cause no increase in congenital malformations, early pregnancy loss, or obstetric complications.[34] Nevertheless, uncertainty remains and concomitant tobacco use is harmful, so any advice should be to reduce levels of use as much as possible during pregnancy.

Conclusion

Whilst abstinence may be best for the fetus, it is frequently an unrealistic objective. Judgmental attitudes by healthcare professionals are inappropriate and unhelpful and drug-using women should be given balanced information that is not unduly alarmist. In view of the potentially high-risk pregnancies, their care should be medically led, but much of it can be delivered by midwives in the community. Management should address social as well as medical problems, and should be provided by a multidisciplinary team in line with national guidelines.[35]

References

1 Home Office Statistical Bulletin. *Statistics of drug addicts notified to the Home Office, United Kingdom, 1994.* London: HMSO, 1995 (Issue 17/95).
2 Department of Health Statistical Bulletin. *Drug misuse statistics bulletin.* London: Department of Health, 1996, No.24.
3 Darke S. The use of benzodiazepines amongst injecting drug users. *Drug Alc Rev* 1995; **13**: 63–9.
4 Seivewright N, Donmall M, Daly C. Benzodiazepines in the illicit drugs scene: the UK picture and some dilemmas. *Int J Drug Policy* 1993; 4(1): 42–8.
5 Information Services Division. *Drug misuse statistics, Scotland.* Edinburgh: Common Services Agency, 1999.
6 Forsyth AJM, Farquhar D, Gemmell M, Shewan D, Davies JB. The dual use of opioids and temazepam by drug injectors in Glasgow (Scotland). *Drug Alc Depend* 1993; **32**: 277–80.
7 Rementeria JL, Janakammal S, Hollander M. Multiple births in drug addicted women. *Am J Obstet Gynecol* 1975; **122**: 958–60.
8 Bai J, Greenwald E, Caterini H, Kaminetzky H. Drug related menstrual aberrations. *Obstet Gynecol* 1974; **44**: 713–9.
9 Perlmutter J. Heroin addiction and pregnancy. *Obstet Gynecol Surv* 1974; b: 439–46.
10 Naeye RL, Blanc W, Leblanc W, Khatamee MA. Fetal complications of maternal heroin addiction: abnormal growth infections and episodes of stress. *J Pediatr* 1973; **83**: 1055–61.
11 Kandall SR, Albin S, Lowinson J, Berle B, Eidelman AI, Gartner LM. Differential effects of maternal heroin and methadone use on birth weight. *Pediatrics* 1976; **58**: 681–5.
12 Zelson C, Rubio E, Wasserman E. Neonatal narcotic addiction: 10 year observation. *Pediatrics* 1971; **48**: 178–89.
13 Kandall SR, Gaines JJ. Maternal substance use and subsequent sudden infant death syndrome (SIDS) in offspring. *Neurotoxicol Teratol* 1991; b: 235–40.
14 Ward SLD, Schuetz S, Krishna V et al. Abnormal sleeping ventilatory pattern in infants of substance-abusing mothers. *AJDC* 1986; **140**: 1015–20.
15 Zuspan FP, Gumpel JA, Mejia-Zelaya A, Davis R. Fetal stress from methadone withdrawal. *Am J Obstet Gynecol* 1975; **122**: 43–6.
16 Hepburn M. Drugs of Abuse. In: Cockburn F, ed. *Advances in perinatal medicine.* London: Parthenon Publishing, 1997, pp. 120–4.
17 Wilson GS, Desmond MM, Verniaud WM. Early development of infants of heroin addicted mothers. *Am J Dis Child* 1973; **126**: 457–62.
18 Blinick G, Jerez E, Wallach RC. Methadone maintenance, pregnancy, and progeny. *JAMA* 1973; b: 477–9.
19 Pierson PS, Howard P, Kleber HD. Sudden death in infants born to methadone-maintained addicts. *JAMA* 1972; **220**: 1733–4.
20 Hulse GK, Milne DR, English CD, Holman CDJ. Assessing the relationship between maternal opiate use and neonatal mortality. *Addiction* 1998; **93**: 1033–42.
21 Strauss ME, Lessen-Firestone JK, Starr RH Jr, Ostrea EM. Behavior of narcotics addicted newborns. *Child Dev Dec* 1975; **46**: 887–93.

22 Rosenberg L, Mitchell AA, Parsella JL, Parshayan H, Louick C, Shapiro S. Lack of relation of oral clefts to diazepam use during pregnancy. *New Engl J Med* 1983; **309**: 1282–5.

23 Bracken MB, Holford TR. Exposure to prescribed drugs in pregnancy and association with congenital malformations. *Obstet Gynaecol* 1981; **58**: 336–44.

24 Laegreid L, Olegard R, Walstrom J, Conradi N. Teratogenic effects of benzodiazepine use during pregnancy. *J Paediat* 1989; **114**: 123–31.

25 Bingol N, Fuchs M, Diaz V, Stone RK, Gromisch DS. Teratogenicity of cocaine in humans. *J Pediatr* 1987; **110**: 93–6.

26 Chasnoff IJ, Burns WJ, Schnoll SH, Burns KA. Cocaine use in pregnancy. *New Engl J Med* 1985; **313**: 666–9.

27 Acker D, Sachs BP, Tracey KJ, Wise WE. Abruptio placentae associated with cocaine use. *Am J Obstet Gynecol* 1983; **146**: 220–1.

28 Chouteau M, Brickner Namerow P, Leppert P. The effect of cocaine abuse on birthweight and gestational age. *Obstet Gynecol* 1988; **72**: 351–4.

29 Zuckerman B, Frank DA, Hingson R et al. Effect of maternal marijuana and cocaine use on fetal growth. *New Engl J Med* 1989; **320**: 762–8.

30 Oro AS, Dixon SD. Perinatal cocaine and methamphetamine exposure: maternal and neonatal correlates. *J Pediatr* 1987; **111**: 571–8.

31 Chasnoff IJ, Burns KA, Burns WJ. Cocaine use in pregnancy: perinatal morbidity and mortality. *Neurotoxicol Teratol* 1987; **9**: 291–3.

32 Hoyme HE, Jones KL, Dixon SD et al. Prenatal cocaine exposure and fetal vascular disruption. *Pediatrics* 1990; **85**: 743–7.

33 Koren G, Graham K, Shear H, Einarson T. Bias against the null hypothesis: the reproductive hazards of cocaine. *Lancet* 1989; **2**: 1440–2.

34 Fried P. Marijuana and human pregnancy. In: Chasnoff IJ, ed. *Drug use in pregnancy: mother and child.* Norwell, Ma: MTP Press, 1986, pp. 64–74.

35 Local Government Drugs Forum (LGDF), Standing Conference on Drug Abuse (SCODA). *Drug using parents: policy guidelines for inter-agency working.* London: LGA, 1997.

13 Prescribing for the pregnant traveller

PAULINE A HURLEY

Key points

- Immunization should only be given in pregnancy if there is a clear indication and travel to an endemic area cannot be avoided.

- No drug regimen ensures complete protection against malaria.

- Women with severe or unstable pre-existing medical problems or a poor past obstetric history should be advised against long distance travel.

Introduction

Prescriptions which need to be considered for the pregnant traveller are immunizations prior to travel, drugs which may be taken for travel sickness, malaria prophylaxis and the treatment of traveller's diarrhoea. This article aims to give an overview of the above and suggestions for the pregnant traveller's "first aid kit"

Immunizations

No vaccine, toxoid or immunoglobulin can be regarded as entirely safe in pregnancy. Acute illness, either as a result of giving a vaccine[1] or as a result of contracting an infection, brings with it the risk of premature labour, with its consequent morbidity and mortality, or the risk of *in-utero* infection. Immunization should only be given in pregnancy if there is a clearly defined risk and travel to endemic areas cannot be avoided.

Box 13.1 summarizes the guidelines for immunization in pregnancy and Table 13.1 gives the current recommendations for travel, derived for the HMSO publication on immunization against infectious disease.

Box 13.1 Guidelines for immunization in pregnancy: possibility of harm in pregnancy

- **There would appear to be no adverse effects outside the first trimester.** Animal studies have not demonstrated a fetal risk but no controlled studies in women:

  - Hepatitis A   immune globulin
  - Rabies   immune globulin
  - Varicella zoster   immune globulin
  - Hepatitis B   immune globulin
  - Tetanus   immune globulin

- **Should only be given if there is a proper indication and risk of infection.** Animal studies have not demonstrated an adverse effect but there are no studies in women:

  - BCG   vaccine
  - Diphtheria   toxoid
  - Influenza   vaccine
  - Plague   vaccine
  - Polio   vaccine
  - Tularaemia   vaccine
  - Cholera   vaccine
  - *E. coli*   vaccine
  - Meningitis   vaccine
  - Pneumococcus   vaccine
  - Tetanus   toxoid
  - Typhoid   vaccine

- The benefits of vaccination may be acceptable. There is positive evidence of fetal risk:

  - Yellow fever   vaccine

- The vaccine is contraindicated in pregnancy:

  - Measles   vaccine
  - Mumps   vaccine
  - Rubella   vaccine
  - Smallpox   vaccine
  - Varicella   vaccine

Table 13.1   Current recommendations for immunization and travel

Area of the world	Recommended for all areas	Recommended for some areas
Indian subcontinent	Hepatitis A Polio Tetanus Typhoid TB	Yellow fever Meningococcal meningitis
Far East	Cholera Hepatitis A Tetanus Polio TB	Japanese encephalitis
Middle East	Hepatitis A Tetanus Polio TB	Meningococcal meningitis
Africa	Cholera Hepatitis A Typhoid Tetanus TB	Yellow fever Meningococcal meningitis Polio
Central and South America	Cholera Hepatitis A TB Typhoid Tetanus Polio	Yellow fever
Eastern Europe	Hepatitis A Polio Tetanus	
Areas out of immediate medical attention or rural stays > 30 days	Rabies Hepatitis B	

Cholera

It should be noted that The World Health Organisation (WHO) no longer recommends cholera vaccination for international travellers and it should no longer be an entry requirement into any foreign country.[2] The vaccine is not effective in that it only provides limited personal protection and does not prevent the spread of this waterborne acute diarrhoeal disease.

Diphtheria

Widespread immunization against diphtheria in childhood has virtually eliminated this disease from the UK but diphtheria toxoid is recommended if neither booster nor immunization has been given in the previous 10 years, and travel to a high risk area (Africa or the Indian subcontinent) cannot be avoided.

Tetanus

Tetanus contracted during pregnancy is associated with high morbidity, with neonatal tetanus mortality being in the region of 65%.[3] There appear to be no adverse effects from giving toxoid in pregnancy, and the American College of Obstetricians and Gynecologists endorse its use in pregnancy, particularly if the woman may deliver in unhygienic circumstances.[4]

Meningitis

At present there is no effective vaccine against the B serogroup of the meningococcus which is the commonest cause of meningitis in the UK.[2] A vaccine is available as a purified bacterial capsular polysaccharide mix of serogroups A and C, but this is only recommended if there is a true risk of infection. This would apply to those travelling to sub-saharan Africa, Delhi, Nepal, Bhutan, Pakistan, and Haj pilgrims travelling to Saudi Arabia.

Typhoid

There are three vaccines available for the prevention of typhoid:

- A monovalent whole cell vaccine which is heat killed and phenol preserved;
- a typhoid Vi polysaccharide antigen containing Vi antigen from the bacterial capsule;
- an oral live attenuated vaccine.

No data are available on the safety of any of these vaccines in pregnancy; none is 100% effective and they certainly do not provide a substitute for careful hygiene and food preparation.[5]

Hepatitis

The risk of acquiring hepatitis A is no different for the pregnant woman than for any other traveller. Whilst it is usually associated with travel to rural areas in developing countries, it has been reported in tourists travelling to destinations closer to home, and, whilst maternal infection is said not to be associated with perinatal transmission, placental abruption and premature delivery of an infected infant has been reported.[6]

Passive immunization with human normal immunoglobulin (HNIG) is the usual mode of protecting the traveller. It works for up to 4 months and carries no apparent risks in pregnancy. A hepatitis A vaccine is available for active immunization but there are no data available on its safety in pregnancy. Theoretically, as it is not a live vaccine, the risk is small, but there are concerns regarding its use in pregnancy, as a febrile response to vaccination is not uncommon.[4]

Hepatitis B infection in pregnancy can cause severe disease in the mother and chronic infection in the neonate.[7] All pregnant women in this country are screened at the beginning of pregnancy and, if they are found to be negative by serology for past infection or immunization, they can be given recombinant hepatitis B vaccine in the unlikely event that they will be travelling to endemic areas and risk exposure to blood or blood products.[4]

Yellow Fever

Yellow fever is spread by the infected mosquito, but confined to tropical Africa and South America. During epidemics, fatality for unimmunized adults can exceed 50%. The vaccine is a live attenuated freeze-dried vaccine. The risks to the fetus are unknown and it should be regarded as contraindicated in pregnancy. There may be circumstances, however, when the risks of the disease outweigh the risk of immunization. Travel to areas requiring documentary evidence of immunization should therefore be avoided in pregnancy.[1]

The areas of greatest risk of exposure to the above diseases are the Far and Middle East, Central and South America, Asia and Eastern Europe and travel to these areas is best avoided in pregnancy.

Malaria prophylaxis

No drug regimen ensures complete protection against malaria. Complications of the disease are more severe in pregnancy, and mid-trimester abortion, preterm delivery and low birthweight are direct complications.[7] Transplacental transmission can occur with devastating consequences for the neonate. Dehydration, thrombocytopenia, splenic rupture, and seizures have all been reported. There is also evidence that placental malarial infection may increase the risk of transmission of other bloodborne pathogens such as HIV.[8]

Avoidance of mosquito bites by physical means is the best advice. This will include the wearing of protective clothing (trousers and long-sleeved shirts), together with the use of insect repellents. Many preparations contain DEET (^{14}C-*N,N*,diethyl-*m*-tolumide), which has been shown to be absorbed through the skin and to cross the placental barrier in some animal studies.[9] The safety of DEET in pregnancy is not established. There is evidence that it accumulates in fatty tissues and brain, and there is a report of a child with mental retardation, impaired sensorimotor coordination, and craniofacial dysmorphology, born to a mother who had applied DEET daily throughout her pregnancy.[10]

It is important to stress that any drug or combination of drugs used for malaria prophylaxis needs to be commenced 1 week before entry and for a further 4 weeks after the malarial area has been left. **Chloroquine** (300 mg weekly) is regarded as safe in pregnancy, but single agent therapy is becoming less effective, and the drug should normally be given in combination with proguanil 200 mg/day, together with folic acid 5 mg/day.[11]

Mefloquine (in a dose of 250 mg/week) is not recommended by the manufacturers for use in the first trimester, but actually appears to be safe in pregnancy, although it is still being monitored.[12] In trials of mefloquine there was a suggestion of an increase in the number of stillbirths, but this was not substantiated in further work.[13,14]

Quinine has been associated with stillbirth and congenital abnormality, but still has a place in the treatment of severely infected pregnant women with falciparum malaria.[15]

Table 13.2 outlines the combinations that have been recommended and comments on their use in pregnancy.

The areas which carry the highest risk of multidrug-resistant malaria are East Africa, Thailand, Papua New Guinea, and the Thai–Cambodia and Myanmar borders. Women should be strongly advised against travelling to these areas during pregnancy.

Antibiotics and other anti-infective agents

Bacterial, viral , fungal, and parasitic infections are not uncommon in pregnancy, with urinary tract infections being a particular risk, and the drugs suitable for the treatment of these conditions are discussed in Chapter 3. Antibiotics may be carried as part of a first-aid kit for travellers, and in general the following may be considered for this purpose:

Table 13.2 Malaria prophylaxis in pregnancy

Drug	Advice in pregnancy	Comments
Chloroquine	Safe in pregnancy	
Proguanil	Safe but recommend folate supplements	May be used in combination with chloroquine
Mefloquine	Appears safe but still being monitored	Reports of tertatogenicity in animal studies
Fansidar	No longer recommended for malaria prophylaxis	Acute skin reactions including Steven–Johnson syndrome and toxic epidermal necrolysis
Maloprim (pyrimethamine and dapsone)	Not recommended in pregnancy	Possible teratogenic risk plus neonatal haemolysis
Doxycycline	Not recommended in pregnancy	
Cinchona alkaloids (quinine and quinidine)	Not used for prophylaxis	Still have a place in the treatment of severe infections

- Amoxycillin for urinary and respiratory infections.
- Metronidazole, a useful antiparasitic, particularly for the treatment of giardiasis and amoebiasis. Whilst it can be used for traveller's diarrhoea it should probably not be carried in a first-aid kit to be administered without medical supervision. It should only be used when other therapeutic options are not available.[16]
- Nystatin and canestan can be safely used topically in pregnancy and should be part of the "kit", particularly in hot climates where the incidence of vaginal candidiasis may be increased.[17]

An overview of the commonly used drugs for the treatment of traveller's diarrhoea and comments relating to their use in pregnancy is given in Table 13.3.[18]

Women taking other regular medications

In general women taking other prescribed medications should be advised that all medications should be taken in their original containers, and to ensure that there are no restrictions on taking them out of the country.

Table 13.3 Drugs used for traveller's diarrhoea in pregnancy

Drug	Indication	Advice in pregnancy
Bismuth subsalycilate (Pepto-Bismuth)		Avoid
Loperamide (Imodium)	Watery diarrhoea	Limited data, but probably safe
Diphenylate with Atropine (Lomotil)	Watery diarrhoea	Use loperamide in preference
Piperazine (Antepar)	Antiparasitic	Contraindicated
Ciprofloxacin	Anti-infective	Safety not yet established
Metronidazole	Giardiasis/amoebiasis	Use only if other therapeutic options not available
Quinacrine	Giardiasis	Contraindicated

Those women with severe or unstable pre-existing disease or who have a poor past obstetric history should be advised against long distance travel, particularly to areas where medical attention may not be readily available.

All travellers should be advised to take with them a first-aid kit that should include a sterile medical pack containing sterile syringes and needles which can be bought over the counter at most good pharmacies. The author's suggestions for the contents of the first aid-kit are shown in Table 13.4.

Table 13.4 Suggestions for a pregnant traveller's first-aid kit

Indication	Suggestion
General	Sterile medical pack
Travel sickness	Vitamin B6 or cyclizine
Malaria Prophylaxis	Chloroquine, proguanil and folic acid
Diarrhoea	Loperamide (and metronidazole for use under medical supervision)
Thrush	Canestan pessary and cream
Urinary tract or upper respiratory tract infection	Amoxycillin
Analgesic	Paracetamol and codeine phosphate

References

1 Hurley P. Vaccination in pregnancy. *Curr Obstet Gynaecol* 1998; **8**: 169–75.
2 Salisbury D, Begg N (eds). Cholera. *Immunisation against infectious disease.* Department of Health, London: HMSO, 1996.
3 Salisbury D, Begg N (eds). Tetanus. *Immunisation against infectious disease.* Department of Health, London: HMSO, 1996.
4 Samuel BU, Barry M. The pregnant traveller. *Infect Dis Clin N Amer* 1998; **12**: 325–54.
5 Salisbury D, Begg N (eds). Typhoid. *Immunisation against infectious disease.* Department of Health, London: HMSO, 1996.
6 Watson JC, Fleming DW, Bordella AJ *et al.*. Vertical transmission of hepatitis A resulting in an outbreak in a neonatal intensive care unit. *J Infect Dis* 1993; **167**: 567–71.
7 Nelson-Piercy C (ed.) *Handbook of obstetric medicine.* Oxford: Isis Medical Media, 1997, p. 162.
8 Bloland PB, Wirima JT, Steketree RW *et al.* Maternal HIV infection and infant mortality in Malawi: Evidence for increased mortality due to placental malaria. *AIDS* 1995; **9**: 721–6.
9 Blomquist L, Thorsell W. Distribution and fate of insect repellent ^{14}C-*N,N* diethyl-*m*-tolumide in the animal: Distribution and excretion after cutaneous application. *Acta Pharmacol Toxicol* 1977; **41**: 235.
10 Sheafer C, Peters PW. Intrauterine diethyltoluamide exposure and fetal outcome. *Reprod Toxicol* 1992; **6**(20): 175–6.
11 Radloff PD, Phillips J, Nkeyi M *et al.* Atovaquone and proguanil for *Plasmodium falciparum* malaria. *Lancet* 1996; **347**: 1511–14.
12 Anonymous. Mefloquine and malaria prophylaxis. *Drug Therapeut Bull* 1998; **36**: 20–2.
13 Nosten F, ter Kuile F, Maelankiri L *et al.* Mefloquine prophylaxis prevents malaria during pregnancy: A double-blind, placebo controlled-study. *J Infect Dis* 1994; **169**: 595–603.
14 Phillips-Howard PA, Steffen R, Kerr L *et al.* Safety of mefloquine nd other antimalarial agents in the first trimester of pregnancy. *J Travel Med* 1998; **5**(3): 121–6.
15 McEvoy GK. Litvak K, Welsh OH *et al* (eds). *American Hospital Formulary Service Drug Information.* Bethesda: American Society of Health – System Pharmacists, 1997.
16 Hammill HA. Metronidazole, clindamycin and quinolones *Obstet Gynecol Clin N Amer* 1989; **16**: 531–40.
17 Rosa FW, Baum C, Shaw M. Pregnancy outcomes after first-trimester vaginitis drug therapy. *Obstet Gynecol* 1987; **69**: 751–5.
18 Hurley PA. Travelling in pregnancy. *The Diplomate* 1999; **5**: 254.

14 Drugs in breastfeeding

JANE M RUTHERFORD

Introduction

Drugs given to a breastfeeding mother may affect her baby. The drugs which have adverse effects on a breastfeeding infant may be different from those which cause problems in pregnancy since the mechanisms of transfer of compounds across the breast differ from those in the placenta. The most important factor is not necessarily whether the drug crosses into breast milk, but the concentration of drug that is present in the neonatal blood and the effect that this might have.

As with the use of drugs during pregnancy, drug companies are generally unwilling to recommend the use of drugs during lactation, because of problems with litigation and the ethical impossibility of performing randomized trials. Therefore, the information available about the effects on infants of drugs given to breastfeeding women is accumulated through case reports and series of various size. Because of this, there is more information and experience regarding older drugs and relatively little about new compounds.

General principles

Maternal drug concentration

The obvious factors which affect maternal drug concentrations are drug dose, frequency, route of administration, and patient compliance. Within two weeks of delivery, the majority of the physiological changes in the circulation that occur as part of pregnancy have reverted to the non-pregnant state. This means that in the first 2 weeks of lactation the plasma concentrations of drugs may vary considerably. Subsequent to this, plasma levels of water-soluble drugs will be similar to those in non-pregnant women. The changes in body fat distribution take longer to revert to the prepregnant state. This results in the plasma concentrations of fat-soluble drugs tending to be lower during lactation than in the non-pregnant state.

Drug transfer across the breast

Most drugs will pass into breast milk in greater or lesser amounts. The amount of drug available for transfer across the breast will depend on blood flow to the breast. It is known that blood flow to the breast increases generally during lactation, but it is not clear whether there are variations in the blood flow during or between feeds.[1] Whether the drug molecules pass across the breast into the milk will then depend on the properties of the drug itself. Small molecules get into breast milk more easily than large ones. Fat-soluble, lipophilic drugs will pass across the cell membrane more easily than those with low lipid solubility. The degree of ionization of the drug and the relative pH of maternal plasma and breast milk also play a role, as does the relative affinity of the drug binding to milk and plasma proteins. In a few instances, active transport mechanisms across the breast have been detected.[1] In addition, there are some drugs that may be metabolized within the breast tissue and metabolites excreted into the milk.[2]

Drug concentration in the infant

One of the factors determining how much drug a baby will ingest is the timing of feeds in relation to maternal dose schedule. The frequency, volume and duration of feeds is also important (Figure 14.1). The milk produced at the beginning of a feed (the foremilk) is protein rich and has a lower fat content to that at the end of a feed (the hindmilk). Therefore, there will be higher concentrations of fat-soluble drugs in the hindmilk. Babies who feed for longer will get increased amounts of such fat soluble compounds compared to those who feed little and often.[2] Infant metabolism is immature compared to adults. Because of this, the half-life of some drugs in the neonatal circulation is longer than in the maternal blood. This may lead to accumulation of drug in the infant.

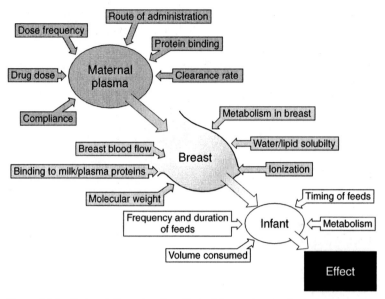

Figure 14.1 Factors influencing the effect of drugs given to the lactating mother on her infant.

Specific agents

The following text and tables (Tables 14.1–14.4) are by no means intended to be comprehensive, but the author has included many of the commonly prescribed drugs. In general, new drugs are to be avoided because of the likely lack of information regarding their safety. The information used in compiling these sections, except where specified, is gathered from references.[1,3-8]

Antimicrobial agents

Any antimicrobial agent which is excreted into breast milk may cause an alteration in the infant's bowel flora and may thus cause diarrhoea. In addition, if the infant develops a pyrexia, it is important that maternal antimicrobial therapy is taken into account.

Analgesic drugs

Paracetamol is excreted into breast milk in very low concentrations, too small to have any effect on the infant, and is therefore the safest analgesic available. Aspirin and salicylates are excreted into breast milk in low concentrations. However, because of immature

Table 14.1 Antimicrobials and breastfeeding

Drug	Comments	Effect on infant	Safety
Penicillin	Low concentrations in breast milk	No specific adverse effects	Safe
Cephalosporins	Low concentrations in breast milk	No specific adverse effects	Safe
Erythromycin	Excreted in breast milk	No specific adverse effects	Safe
Azithromycin	No data	No specific adverse effects	Safe
Tetracyclines	Low concentrations in breast milk	Theoretical risk of tooth discolouration and disruption of bone growth. Unlikely in reality because of low infant serum concentration	Avoid if possible
Sulphonamides	Low concentrations in breast milk	Risk of kernicterus in preterm, ill, or stressed infants	Safe in healthy term infants. Avoid in preterm, ill, or stressed neonates
Aminoglycosides	Present in breast milk and may be absorbed by infant in small amounts, but absorption from GI tract poor	No specific data	Benefits probably outweigh risk
Metronidazole	Excreted into breast milk	Gives breast milk an unpleasant taste	Probably safe
Ciprofloxacin	Excreted into breast milk	Little human data	Avoid because of lack of data. Allow 48 hours after last dose before resuming feeding
Chloramphenicol	Excreted into breast milk	Potential risk of bone-marrow suppression. Concentrations too low to cause the grey baby syndrome	Avoid
Acyclovir	Concentrated in breast milk. Levels exceed those in maternal serum	No adverse effects identified	Probably safe, particularly as it is used to treat herpes virus infections in the neonate with no adverse effects
Antimalarial drugs	Excreted in low concentrations not high enough to provide antimalarial protection to the infant	No adverse effects with the older drugs (*chloroquine*, *proguanil*). Little data about *mefloquine*	*Chloroquine* and *proguanil* are considered safe. Avoid *mefloquine* because of lack of data
Antituberculosis drugs	Excreted in low concentrations	No adverse effects with *ethambutol* and *rifampicin*. No data on *pyrazinamide*. Theoretical risk of interference with nucleic acid function and hepatotoxicity with *isoniazid* but no adverse reactions reported	Probably safe

Table 14.2 Antihypertensives and other cardiovascular drugs

Drug	Comments	Effect on infant	Safety
Hydralazine	Excreted in breast milk	No reported adverse effects	Considered safe
Nifedipine[10]	Low concentrations in breast milk	No reported adverse effects	Considered safe
Methyldopa[11]	Excreted into breast milk in small amounts	No reported adverse effects	Considered safe
Beta-blockers			
Propranolol Labetalol	Excreted into breast milk	No reports of adverse effects but theoretical risk of respiratory depression, bradycardia, and hypoglycaemia	Beta-blockers are probably safe in conjunction with breastfeeding. Infants should be observed for signs of beta-blockade. It has been suggested that atenolol and metoprolol be avoided because of the high concentrations in milk.[13,14] However, there has been extensive use of atenolol with only one report of an adverse event and the risks are probably minimal
Metoprolol Atenolol	Concentrated in breast milk[12,13]	One report of features of beta-blockade in infant where mother was taking atenolol[13]	
Thiazide diuretics	Low concentrations in breast milk	Large doses may suppress lactation	Safe in normal doses
Frusemide	Low concentrations in breast milk	No reports of adverse effects	Safe
Captopril Enalapril	Amounts in breast milk negligible	No reports of adverse effects	Probably safe
Amiodarone	Contains iodine. Excreted into breast milk. Long half-life in adults – unknown in neonates	Few data on infant effects	Avoid during breastfeeding. Do not commence breastfeeding if the mother has taken amiodarone for prolonged periods within the preceding few months
Digoxin	Excreted into breast milk	No reports of adverse effects	Probably safe

Table 14.3   Hormones and drugs used for endocrine conditions

Drug	Comments	Effect on infant	Safety
Insulin	Does not pass into breast milk	None	Safe
Metformin	No reports located regarding passage into breast milk	No reports located and therefore effects unknown	
Chlorpropamide/ tolbutamide	Excreted into breast milk	No reports of adverse effects but hypoglycaemia is a potential risk	Use only with caution
Thyroxine	Low concentrations in breast milk	Concentrations not high enough to protect the infant from neonatal hypo-thyroidism. May interfere with diagnosis of hypothyroidism on Guthrie test	Safe
Carbimazole/ methimazole	Excreted into breast milk	Theoretical risk of thyroid suppression. Evidence suggests that if < 15 mg/day is given to the mother then there is no effect on the infant	Lowest effective dose should be given. Monitor infant thyroid function weekly
Propylthiouracil	Low concentrations in breast milk	No reports of adverse effects	Probably safe. Monitor infant thyroid function
Radioactive iodine (I^{131})	Concentrated in breast milk	Can be taken up by infant thyroid and result in permanent thryoid damage	Contraindicated
Combined oral contraceptive pill	Oestrogen enters breast milk in concentrations less than physiological levels	No effect on infant but may shorten duration of lactation	Avoid because of effects on lactation
Progestogen-only pill		No effect	Safe
Androgens/ antiandrogens	Pass into breast milk	May cause androgenic/antiandrogenic effects on infant	Contraindicated
Danazol		May cause androgenic effects on infant	Contraindicated

Table 14.4 Antipsychotic drugs, antidepressants and sedatives

Drug	Comments	Effect on infant	Safety
Phenothiazines (chlorpromazine, flupenthixol, haloperidol)	Excreted into breast milk	Few data but may cause drowsiness and lethargy. Theoretical effects of dopamine receptor antagonism on the developing central nervous system	No evidence to discontinue breastfeeding but caution should be exercised
Lithium	Excreted into breast milk in significant concentrations	No adverse effects reported but potential for toxicity is high. No studies of long-term effects	Use only with caution. Controlling maternal drug levels will help to minimize risks. Observe infant for signs of toxicity
Tricyclic antidepressants (amytriptyline, imipramine, desipramine)	Excreted into breast milk	Negligible concentrations detected in infant serum. No adverse effects reported	Probably safe but exercise some caution
Doxepin	Excreted into breast milk	Metabolites may accumulate in infant serum. One report of respiratory depression	Avoid if possible
Fluoxetine, sertraline, paroxetine	Excreted into breast milk	One report of irritability and colic in infant. Long-term effects have not been studied. Concerns exist about the unknown effects on neurobehaviour and development	Uncertain safety profile
Diazepam	Excreted into breast milk	May accumulate in the infant and lead to sedation. Withdrawal may also cause adverse effects	Avoid
Temazepam	Excreted into breast milk	No adverse effects reported but risk of sedative effect if large doses given	Use only with caution. Avoid breastfeeding if large amounts taken as drug of abuse

metabolism, high concentrations could potentially accumulate in infant serum which may theoretically result in platelet dysfunction and Reye's syndrome. There is, however, only one report in the literature of salicylate toxicity in a breastfed infant despite its extensive use. In view of the theoretical risks, analgesic doses of aspirin should probably be avoided since other agents are available. Where low dose aspirin is used as thromboprophylaxis, then breastfeeding is probably safe.

There are no reports of adverse effects with the NSAIDs diclofenac, ibuprofen, mefenamic acid, and naproxen, which are all excreted into breast milk in very low concentrations and are therefore safe during lactation. Although there was a single case of neonatal seizures in association with indomethacin,[9] no further such events have been identified and it is therefore probably safe.

Opiates

Morphine is excreted into breast milk. It is unlikely to cause adverse effects in therapeutic doses. However, because of the immature infant metabolism, the half-life is prolonged and accumulation of the drug can occur. Pethidine and its active metabolite are excreted into breast milk. The half-lives are much longer in infants than in adults because of immature metabolism. Repeated doses, particularly in patient-controlled analgesia devices may lead to accumulation and cause neurobehavioural depression. Caution should therefore be exercised. Fentanyl and alfentanyl are safe to use in breastfeeding as the concentration in breast milk is negligible. Codeine passes into breast milk in concentrations that are of minimal significance, and it is therefore safe in breastfeeding.

Anticoagulant drugs

Heparin, because of its large molecular weight, is not excreted into breast milk. Warfarin is also not excreted into breast milk. Both of these agents are therefore safe for use in breastfeeding. There is little information on the effects of low molecular weight heparins, such as dalteparin and enoxaparin, on breastfed infants. However, there are unlikely to be any adverse effects since they have relatively high molecular weights and probably do not pass into breast milk. In addition, if they were present in the milk they would be inactivated in the infant's gastrointestinal tract. Other oral anticoagulants (for example phenindione) should be avoided. For information on aspirin see under analgesic drugs.

Anti-asthmatic drugs

There are few data available on the effects of beta-agonist drugs, such as salbutamol and terbutaline, particularly when taken by inhalation. However, no adverse reports have been located and, in view of the extent of the use of such drugs in women of child-bearing age, it is likely that if adverse effects existed, they would have been detected. These drugs are therefore probably safe.

Theophylline is excreted into breast milk in low concentrations. There is one report of irritability in an infant following ingestion of a rapidly absorbed aminophylline solution. Young infants may experience toxicity at lower levels than older infants. Slow release preparations are therefore more likely to be well tolerated and caution should be exercised.

There are no reports of the effects of inhaled steroids on breastfed infants. However, since oral corticosteroids are considered safe, inhaled steroids are also probably safe.

Antihistamines

There are few reports on the effects of antihistamines on breastfed infants.

Antiepileptic drugs

Phenytoin, carbamazepine, and sodium valproate are excreted into breast milk. There is little risk to the neonate if drug levels in the mother are maintained within the therapeutic range. They are considered safe.

Phenobarbitone is excreted in breast milk and, because of immature infant metabolism, can accumulate in the infant. This can result in sedation. Withdrawal effects have also been observed after abrupt withdrawal of breastfeeding in a woman taking phenobarbitone. Breastfeeding should therefore be avoided if possible.

Lamotrigine is excreted into the breast milk. A recent report suggests that the concentrations of the drug in the infant are minimal.[15] There are no reports of adverse effects in breastfed infants of mothers taking lamotrigine; however, it is a relatively new drug and caution should therefore be exercised.

There is no information about the effects of gabapentin or vigabatrin in breastfeeding.

Gastrointestinal drugs

Drugs affecting gastric acid Simple antacids are generally considered to be safe during breastfeeding. Cimetidine and

187

ranitidine[16] are actively transported into breast milk with high milk: plasma ratios. However, the dose received by the infant is lower than that given to treat infant problems. There are no reports of adverse effects and they are therefore probably safe. There are no data available on the transfer of omeprazole into human milk, or its effects on breastfeeding infants. It is a potent drug which could affect the secretion of gastric acid by the infant. Because of the lack of data it should be avoided if possible.

Laxatives Laxative drugs that are absorbed from the maternal gastrointestinal tract may pass into the breast milk and cause diarrhoea in the infant. If laxatives are necessary, it is preferable to prescribe bulk laxatives, such as ispaghula husk, that are not absorbed.

Antiemetics Prochlorperazine is probably secreted into breast milk. There are no data regarding adverse effects. There is also no information regarding cyclizine. However, since there are no reports of adverse effects with these drugs, and they have been available for a considerable time, they are probably safe. Metoclopramide is concentrated in breast milk. However, the total daily dose received by a breastfed infant of a mother receiving 30 mg/day is less than the dose recommended for therapeutic use in infants or premature neonates. The only adverse effects reported are two cases of mild abdominal discomfort. Although it is probably safe, caution should be exercised because of the theoretical central nervous system effects.

Drugs for inflammatory bowel disease Mesalazine, suphasalazine, and olsalazine are excreted in low concentrations into breast milk. Diarrhoea that resolved on stopping the drug has occurred in the infants of breastfeeding mothers taking these compounds. However, other adverse effects have not been reported. These drugs are not contraindicated, but caution should be taken when these drugs are prescribed in breastfeeding, and the infants should be observed carefully for changes in stool consistency.

Immunosuppressants

Prednisolone is excreted into the breast milk in small quantities.[17] It has been used extensively in breastfeeding women and there have been no reports of serious adverse effects. It is therefore considered safe.

188

Gold is excreted into breast milk and is absorbed by the infant. Adverse effects in infants such as rashes, nephritis, hepatitis, and haematological abnormalities have been reported but a causal relationship not established. However, there is the potential for toxicity in the infant and caution should be exercised.

There are few data regarding other immunosuppressant drugs such as azathioprine, methotrexate, cyclophosphamide, and cyclosporin. However, because of the high potential toxicity of these drugs, they should probably be avoided in breastfeeding, or lactation discontinued.

References

1 Wilson JT, Brown RD, Cherek DR *et al*. Drug excretion in human breast milk: principles, pharmacokinetics and projected consequences. *Clin Pharmacokinet* 1980; **5**: 1–66.
2 Wilson JT, Hinson JL, Brown D, Smith IJ. A comprehensive assessment of drugs and toxins in breast milk. In: Hamosh M, Goldman AS eds. *Human lactation 2: maternal and environmental factors*. New York: Plenum press, 1986.
3 Bennet PN. *The WHO working group. Drugs and human lactation: a guide to the content and consequences of drugs, micronutrients, radiopharmaceuticals and environmental and occupational chemicals in human milk*. Amsterdam: Elsevier Science publishers BV, 1988.
4 Briggs GG, Freeman RK, Yaffe SJ. *Drugs in pregnancy and lactation*. Baltimore: Williams and Wilkins, 1998.
5 Committee on Drugs. The transfer of drugs and other chemicals into human milk. *Pediatrics* 1994; **93**: 137–50.
6 Lee JJ, Rubin AP. Breast feeding and anaesthesia. *Anaesthesia* 1993; **48**: 616–25.
7 Pons G, Rey E, Matheson I. Excretion of psychoactive drugs into breast milk. *Clin Pharmacokinet* 1994; **27**: 270–89.
8 Smith IJ, Wilson JT. Infant effects of drugs excreted into breast milk. *Pediat Rev Commun* 1989; **3**: 93–113.
9 Eeg-Olofsson O, Malmros I, Elwin CE, Steen B. Convulsions in a breast-fed infant after maternal indomethacin. *Lancet* 1978; **2**: 215.
10 Ehrenkranz RA, Ackerman BA, Hulse JD. Nifedipine transfer into human milk. *J Pediatr* 1989; **114**: 478–80.
11 White WB, Andreoli JW, Cohn RD. Alpha-methyl dopa disposition in mothers with hypertension and in their breast fed infants. *Clin Pharmacol Ther* 1985; **37**; 387–90.
12 Liedholm H, Melander A, Bitzen P-O *et al*. Accumulation of atenolol and metoprolol in human breast milk. *Eur J Clin Pharmacol* 1981; **20**: 229–31.
13 Schmimmel MS, Eidelman AJ, Wilschanski MA, Shaw D, Ogilvie RJ, Koren G. Toxic effects of atenolol consumed during breast feeding. *J Pediatr* 1989; **114**: 476–8.
14 Anderson PO. Letter. *Pediatrics* 1995; **95**: 957.
15 Rambeck B, Kurleman G, Stodieck SRG, May TW, Jurgens U. Concentrations of lamotrigine in a mother on lamotrigine treatment and her newborn child. *Eur J Clin Pharmacol* 1997; **51**: 481–4.
16 Oo CY, Kuhn RJ, Desai N, McNamara PJ. Active transport of cimetidine into human milk. *Clin Pharmacol Ther* 1995; **58**: 548–55.
17 Öst L, Wettrall G, Bjorkhelm I, Rane A. Prednisone excretion in human milk. *J Pediatr* 1985; **106**: 1008–11.

Index

INDEX

192

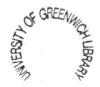